Healthy Easy Cooking

Healthy Kale and Delicious Smoothie Recipes

Sarah Littlefair

Table of Contents

Healthy Easy Cooking Introduction

This book features recipes that help to make a healthy lifestyle, resulting in a strong immune system and maintaining your ideal weight. There are two diets featured here, the Great Kale Recipes diet and the Smoothie Diet. Each diet focuses on including healthy ingredients to create delicious and filling meals with the goal in mind to lose weight and be healthier. Each diet plan features super foods, which are foods packed with vital nutrients that the body needs.

The first section is about the kale diet. In the All About Kale section you will discover why this green leafy vegetable is a super food. You will quickly learn how there can be a whole diet system and even half of this book devoted to this one vegetable. Kale is no longer just a green veggie, often cooked as an afterthought and as a mere side dish. This food is taking center stage and being the star of the meal plan and with good reason.

The second section is about how to store kale. Because it is a fairly delicate vegetable (how long can you store a bag of 'leaves'?) you need to learn how to handle it and store it. Because kale is at the center of this particular diet, you will be keeping a good supply of it on hand for daily use. By learning how to handle and store it you will have a better time with preparing the recipes in this book. Storage does make a difference so pay attention to this section.

The third section covers kale breakfast recipes. Enjoy favorites such as Wilted Kale, Breakfast Pizza Casserole, Kale Cake Muffins, English Muffin Personal Pizzas, Kale Quiche, Ham and Cheese Pinwheels, Super Green Smoothie, Kale Omelet with Mushrooms and Feta Cheese, Easy Breakfast Casserole, and a tasty Breakfast Burrito. With these great recipes, you may wish to serve them for lunch and supper too and that is okay with us.

The fourth section covers soup recipes featuring kale as the main ingredient. It is no wonder kale is so easy to cook with because it goes so well with so many different foods. It allows other foods to take the lead in the flavor and blends well into the background. Some of the soup recipes include Sri Lanka Kale Coconut Soup, Kale and Avocado Gazpacho, Raw Kale Soup, Green Power Soup, Kale Gazpacho, Dilled Kale, Beets and Tofu Soup, and Sesame Noodle and Kale Soup.

The fifth section covers salad recipes with kale as the

primary ingredient. Because kale is a leafy green vegetable of course, it is perfect in the raw state and makes for a delicious salad green. Try some of these recipes: Kale Salad with Parmesan, Avocado and Apricots, Pickled Watermelon Radish with Kale Salad, Kale Salad with Meyer Lemon and Blood Orange, Kale Slaw with Peanut Dressing, Northern Spy Kale Salad, and Kale Salad with Lemon and Pecorino.

The sixth section is full of using kale as main dish recipes. This gives you more than a couple weeks worth of meals for the Kale Diet. Choose from an assortment of recipes including Kale with Sesame Noodles, Vegetarian Lasagna with Kale, Kale wand Spinach Turnover, White Bean Soup with Chorizo and Kale, Greens and Garbanzo Beans, Garlic Roasted Kale, Kale with Steamed Halibut and Walnuts, Braised Chicken with Kale, and Cajun Chicken Skillet with Kale.

The seventh section is, believe it or not, about using kale as the primary ingredient in desserts. Who says dieting means you have to give up the foods you love? Not on the kale diet, because you get to enjoy desserts such as Pesto and Kale Muffins, Kale Colada, Kale, Pancetta Pie and Butternut Squash, Blueberry Kale Ice cream, Coconut and Chocolate Kale Chips, Parmesan and Kale Scones, Apple and Kale Muffins, and Bacon and Kale

Bread Pudding.

The next sections are about the smoothie diet and learn how this diet can affect you. First, you will find information on smoothies, why they are beneficial, and how you can use them in your diet plan. Smoothies, while easy to fix, do require special equipment and special instructions on preparation. It is an easy plan though, once you learn how to fix the smoothies you will see how super easy this diet is to maintain. With the smoothie diet you will experience a body cleanse as well as lose weight.

Smoothies require certain ingredients. The next section covers this by listing the "main" ingredients that are common to all smoothies. This section also covers the categories that smoothies fall under such as fruit smoothies, green smoothies, breakfast smoothies and energy smoothies. Each of these categories provides smoothies fit either to replace a full meal or to enhance snack time.

One of the major benefits for the smoothie diet is the detoxification it does for the body. In particular, the liver is the one system that receives a good cleansing from ingesting a true smoothie diet, especially if you use the recipes found within this book. Discover how the smoothie diet works in detoxifying the liver and how it can benefit your overall health.

Another benefit and probably the main reason people go on the smoothie diet is to lose weight. It only stands to reason if you go on the smoothie diet you will go through a detoxification, which also results in weight loss. Once the detox is over the weight can continue to fall off, while the highly nutritious smoothies give the body all the nutrients including protein need.

The remaining sections cover the recipes for the smoothie diet including the five-day sample menu plan. Even the five-day menu plan has valuable recipes that go well with the smoothies. Here are a sample of the recipes: The Frozen Banana Smoothie, Nutty Creamy Apple Smoothie, Pumpkin Apple Smoothie with Cinnamon, Pineapple Vanilla Smoothie, Tomatocado, Bell Pepper Avocado Smoothie, Celery Red Grape Smoothie, Plum Banana Smoothie, Basic Sweet Grapefruit Smoothie, Raspberry Peach Smoothie, Coffee Banana Tofu Smoothie, All Day Energy Smoothie, Basic Protein Smoothie, Basic Apricot Breakfast Smoothie, Mango Tomato Smoothie, and the Cocoa Peanut Butter Smoothie.

Section 1: All About Kale: Why is it a Superfood?

There are many foods that are good for the body. Fruits and vegetables are considered to be part of a healthy diet. There are some foods that are known as super foods. They contain a number of vitamins and minerals. In addition to promoting good health they can help with ailments as well. Kale is considered to be one of these super foods. Usually, kale is simply used as a garnish, or thrown in with other collard greens. But, as you'll discover throughout this book, there are far more uses than that.

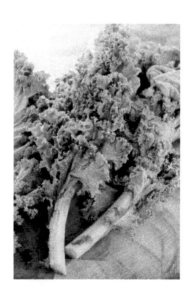

Kale is a vegetable with a high number of nutrients. It is one of the healthiest foods that a person can eat. Kale is in the same vegetable family as broccoli, cabbage, and Brussels sprouts. it is packed with more vitamins per bite than many other vegetables. This vegetable will help keep a person healthy. Kale can even help the body defend itself against cancer. This food can help prevent stomach, colon, breast, and ovarian cancers.

Kale is able to help the body stay healthy by providing the daily values of many different vitamins. Kale is high in vitamin K, vitamin A, and vitamin C. It also contains a significant amount of copper and manganese. Kale has an adequate amount of many other vitamins including vitamin B6, potassium, calcium, thiamin, riboflavin, niacin, zinc, and iron. Kale also contains omega 3 fatty acids which help with memory and brain development.

Kale has many anti-oxidant powers that will keep a person from getting ill, and can help fight off any pre existing illness. Some of the anti-oxidants that can be found in kale include B-carotene, lutein, and zeaxanthin. The carotene will help a person keep their eyes strong and healthy. This vitamin is also said to improve the vision of a person that is having trouble seeing already. One study found that people who ate a lot of kale in their diet were able to reduce their risk of developing cataracts by fifty percent.

Kale is low in calories and these calories are easy for the body to use and to burn. A one cup serving of kale has only 36 calories. This same serving size has 192% of a person's recommended daily amount of Vitamin A. It is said that the body cannot overdose on vitamin A. This same serving of kale is around 90% of the daily value of vitamin C that is recommended for a person to stay healthy. Vitamin C will help prevent cells from being damaged and will help the body repair any cells that are damaged. This vitamin will also help inflammation and help to keep cholesterol at a healthy level. Vitamin C will also help the body fight off colds and other illnesses.

Kale contains trace minerals that help with certain functions of the body. Manganese will help the body burn and use different types of fatty acids. They will also help the acid reach sex cells and the nervous system for use. These minerals will also aid the body in using and burning both proteins and carbohydrates. Kale can help the body burn fat and keep the body for storing new fatty deposits. The amount of calcium that is found in kale will help the body to keep strong bones. It will also help to prevent the onset of osteoporosis. This mineral will also promote the development of collagen in the skin, which will help a person remain youthful in appearance.

Kale is one of the three green and leafy vegetables that can keep a person mentally sharp even as they age. This vegetable will slow the mental decline in a person that comes with old age. Kale alone can slow this mental decline down by 40%. This is similar to reversing the aging process by five years. Kale has many vitamins and minerals that benefit the inside of the body as well. Kale contains a photochemical known as idole-3-carbinol. This biochemical will help lower the amount of secretion from the liver. It also blocks the transfer of the LDL also known as the "bad cholesterol" from entering the tissues in the body and getting into the blood stream. Kale will also help a person burn stubborn belly fat that exercise and diet alone do not get rid of.

With all of these nutrients and vitamins in kale it is a natural fat burner. It is very low in calories and does not contain fat. Kale will help the body with its urinary track systems as well. Kale helps to protect the bladder as well as bladder cancer. Many people that have had urinary tract infections know how painful this can be. Eating kale can help a person from getting this condition. This one again is due to the amount of vitamin A that is found in this leafy vegetable.

In order to get the most health benefits out of kale it should be eaten soon after being purchased. Kale can also be grown in a garden. Kale has a rating of 1,770 on the ORAC scale. This scale is a rating of the amount of antioxidants that are found in food. Other vegetables only have ratings that are in the hundreds. Kale has a rating of at least a thousand more than other vegetables on this scale.

While kale is good for the body it is not the most attractive vegetable to eat. Kale is dark green in color and curly. There are several ways that a person can prepare kale. It can be chopped up while it is raw and added to salads. It can be cooked and included in casseroles, soups, and stir fries. With all the benefits to the body this super food contains, it does not matter how a person eats it. Many of the recipes that contain kale are low in calories and low in fat. Kale provides so many vitamins and minerals, it could be eaten on a daily basis to help a person stay healthy.

How to Store Kale

Kale is the buzz word among busy families looking for an easy to prepare, nutrient-dense food. Kale offers variety from other leafy greens. Whether choosing the younger, tender leaves for intense, flavorful salads, or the more mature leaves for cooking as a side dish of wilted greens, kale is finding a place on more and more tables. As this super food becomes more widely known, people everywhere are asking how to choose it, how to use it, and how best to keep it on hand to enjoy any time.

Kale is a deep green leafy member of the cruciferous family, a relative of broccoli, collards, cabbage, and Brussels sprouts. It is available in several varieties, including curly, the most common, ornamental, and Tuscan, with its longer, more slender leaves.

As with any fresh produce, there are a number of things to consider when choosing Kale at the market for flavor, freshness and optimum storage. First, consider how you will serve it. Larger leaves may be bitter for salads, but will cook well to serve as a side dish of greens. Younger more tender leaves are ideal for salads. Look for strong stems, not limp.

The firm leaves should be a deep green. Avoid signs of yellow or brown leaves or small holes in the leaves. Avoid signs of wilting, which indicate an older product that probably will not store well, and may be more likely to contain contaminants. In fact, you may want to consider choosing an organically raised product, as Kale is a member of the most widely contaminated produce varieties known as "the dirty dozen."

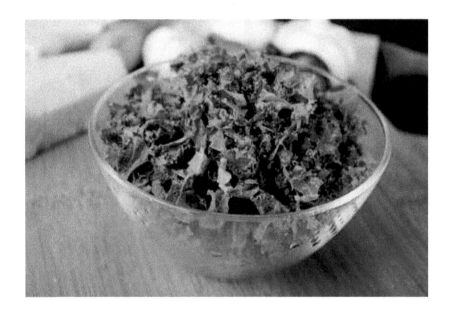

However, it's delicious and nutritious benefits far outweigh any risks, and you should not hesitate to make kale a new and permanent part of your family's diet. Proper preparation and storage is the key. In general, kale can be prepared for storage just as one would prepare it for serving. Whether for use as a salad green or for cooking, it is best to remove the tough stems.

Grab the stem firmly in one hand and with a tight grip of the other hand, pull down and away, stripping the tender leaves from the stem. The leaves themselves will stay fairly well intact. Toss the stems away, and toss the leaves into a cold water bath. Agitate the leaves to remove any grit and soil. Remove the leaves, squeezing out any excess water. From here you can choose to boil the kale and serve it wilted as a side dish, serve it fresh in a salad, or store it to enjoy later.

To store it you may refrigerate it or freeze it. If you are refrigerating, it is very important at this point to get the kale as dry as possible. For this reason, many people prefer to refrigerate it without washing, and clean it as they use it. If you wash it first, blot it as dry as possible with paper towels. Place the kale in sealable plastic bags, removing as much of the air as possible as you seal it. In the coldest part of the refrigerator, it should keep well for 5 to 7 days. Be aware that the leaves will become more bitter, the longer kale is kept. For longer storage, kale can also be frozen. Clean and wash it as described above. Blanch the leaves for 2 minutes in boiling water, and plunge them immediately into an ice water bath. Drain and place the blanched kale in sealable freezer bags, removing as much of the air as possible. Kale can be kept frozen for 10 to 12 months. One advantage of freezing is that frozen kale can tend to have a slightly sweeter taste, not as bitter as fresh.

If kale becomes a regular part of your family's diet, as it has for many, consider growing it yourself. Let nature herself handle the storage for you. The leaves can be harvested for each intended use, young tender leaves for salads, older leaves to be cooked. Just pick as needed and the kale keeps producing so that you can harvest as you go, just as you would with cut and come again lettuces. Kale is a hardy winter vegetable. Frost actually improves its flavor. And you can store it frozen right in the garden to enjoy all winter long. Mature plants will survive right through the toughest winter weather, down to 10°F or below.

Finally, one of the most popular uses for kale lately is in the form of bite-size dehydrated chips. Kale chips are available in health food markets everywhere. They don't stay on the shelves long, and they won't stay in the house long once your family has tasted this trendy new snack. But healthy as they are, delicious kale chips can be expensive. Consider making them yourself at home. There are many easy recipes readily available online, but here is perhaps the simplest. Just tear tender young kale leaves into bite-size pieces, coat in extra-virgin olive oil and sea salt, and spread them out on rimmed baking sheets.

Without an expensive food dehydrator, you can roast them for an hour in a very low oven, 170°F. Turn off the heat and let them rest in the oven another half hour. Then turn the oven back on for another 20 minutes. The result will be crispy delicious salty chips your family or party guests will rave about. Leftover chips will keep well for several days in a brown paper bag. If they become soft, they can be re-crisped in a low oven and served again as fresh as just-made.

Kale is a super food which is growing in popularity. It is easy to find and easy to keep on hand. Whether you enjoy it as a salad, as wilted greens, or as a substitute for your favorite salty snack chip, whether you shop for it at the local market or grow it yourself, you can make kale a delicious new choice for your family's table.

10 Great Kale Recipes: Breakfast

Easy Breakfast Casserole

Ingredients

8 eggs

1/2 cup chopped ham, sausage or bacon bits

1/4 teaspoon salt

1 cup fresh kale, finely chopped

Pinch black pepper

1 cup shredded cheese (white cheddar)

1/4 cup Parmesan cheese

1/2 cup half and half

3 or 4 chopped scallions

Directions

Preheat oven to 350°

Prepare a 9 x 13 inch casserole dish with non-stick cooking spray.

Beat together the black pepper, salt, half and half and eggs.

Mix in kale.

Add ham, sausage or bacon.

Pour the ingredients the casserole dish.

Top casserole with Cheddar and Parmesan cheeses then garnish with chopped scallions.

Bake 30-40 minutes, or until the middle is firm.

Breakfast Burrito

Ingredients

4 large eggs
2 7 ½ inch flour tortillas
2 tablespoons milk
1 tablespoon fresh cilantro (chopped)
1/2 cup fresh chopped kale
2 tablespoons olive oil
1/2 cup grated Pepper Jack or Monterey Jack
Pepper and Salt
2 tablespoons sour cream (optional)

Directions

Preheat the oven to 350°F then place the tortillas in foil, wrap them and place them in oven to warm.

Whisk the pepper, salt, milk, cilantro and eggs in a bowl.

Add olive oil to a skillet (nonstick) over medium-low heat.

Add kale, stirring for about 1 minute then put in eggs and cook, while stirring, until just firm. Spoon eggs along the middle of the tortillas then top with sour cream and cheese. Fold tortilla.

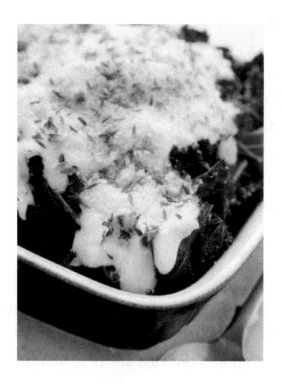

Kale Omelet with Mushrooms and Feta Cheese

Ingredients

Pepper and Salt
1 tablespoon feta cheese
1 teaspoon olive oil
1/4 cup mushroom pieces (fresh)
1 cup fresh kale
2 eggs (beaten)

Directions

Heat oil in a small skillet on med heat then put in mushrooms and kale and sauté until the mushrooms are properly heated and the kale starts to wilt.

Put in eggs. Cook until eggs are firm, lifting the edges to let uncooked part of egg flow to the bottom. Flip if desired.

Add pepper and salt to taste.

Put in feta cheese then, fold in half and serve.

Super Green Smoothie

Ingredients

1 cup fresh kale
1 tablespoon lemon juice
1/4 cup orange juice or water
1/2 cup fresh blueberries
1 banana
4 ice cubes

Directions

Blend together the water/orange juice, blueberries, banana and ice cubes until consistency is smooth. Put in kale and blend again until completely smooth and creamy.

Wilted Kale

Ingredients

1 cup sliced mushrooms
2 cups kale
1 lb bacon

Directions

Fry bacon then put to one side
Put mushrooms and kale in bacon grease then stir over
medium-high heat until well-heated and kale starts to
wilt.

Serve immediately.

Ham and Cheese Pinwheels

Ingredients:

1 packet ranch dressing mix (dry)
4 oz sour cream
4 oz spreadable whipped cream cheese
Fresh kale leaves
4-8 slices deli ham (or turkey ham)
1 can crescent rolls

Directions

Grease cookie sheet. Preheat oven to 400. Then roll the crescent rolls out.

In a bowl, whisk together ranch dressing mix, cream cheese and sour cream.

Spread mixture in a thin layer over the crescents.

Add one slice of ham and one kale leaf to each crescent.

Roll lengthwise then to close the dough pinch the ends.

Bake until golden brown (15-20 minutes).

Let cool for 10 minutes then Cut into bite-sized slices.

Breakfast Pizza Casserole

Ingredients

1 cup grated Cheddar cheese
6 eggs
1/2 cup chopped onion
2 cups shredded kale
1 cup frozen hash brown potatoes (thaw)
1 can crescent dinner rolls
1 lb. ground pork sausage

Directions

Brown sausage in a skillet, then let drain and put to one side.

Unroll the crescent roll into a baking dish that is lightly greased. Press the sides and bottom to make a crust. Use a fork to create several small holes.

Bake crust at 350 degrees on the lower rack in the oven for 5 - 6 minutes. Spoon the over crust evenly then top with kale, onion and potatoes.

Beat eggs and pour mixture over potatoes then bake without covering dish at 350 degrees on until set (approximately 25 minutes) on lower oven rack.

Sprinkle cheese evenly over top then let bake until cheese melts (approximately 5 minutes).

Kale Quiche

Ingredients

Dash black pepper
1/2 tsp. salt
3 slices crumbled cooked bacon
2 beaten eggs
1 cup milk
2 cups cooked kale
2 tablespoons flour
2 cups shredded cheese (sharp cheddar)
1 ready-to-use pie crust (refrigerated)

Directions

Preheat oven to 350°F.

Place crust in a pie plate (9-inch) then flute edge and use a fork to prick.

In medium sized bowl mix flour and cheese then put in remaining ingredients. Pour mixture into crust and let bake for approximately 1 hour.

Kale Cake Muffins

Ingredients

1 1/2 cups flour (all purpose)
1/2 cup unsweetened applesauce
2 tablespoons oil (vegetable)
1 teaspoon powder (baking)
1/3 cup sugar
1 cup fresh kale
2 teaspoons vanilla extract
1/2 teaspoon baking soda
1 large egg
1/2 teaspoon salt

Directions

Preheat the oven to 350 F.

Use a food processor to puree oil, sugar, kale, vanilla, egg and applesauce.

In another bowl mix the dry ingredients.

Pour the puree into a big mixing bow then slowly mix in dry ingredients until well combined.

Place batter in lined or greased mini muffin tin (only fill two thirds of each cup).

Bake 12-15 minutes.

English Muffin Personal Pizzas

Ingredients

1 teaspoon salt
Oregano
Mozzarella (grated)
1/2 cup kale (finely chopped)
2 sliced hard-cooked eggs
Slices of tomato
4 teaspoons olive oil
4 English muffins

Directions

Cut English muffins in half and toast them then place them on a cookie sheet.

Drizzle the olive oil on each one.

Place one slice of tomato on each half of muffin.

Layer on 2 or 3 egg slices

Add desired amount of cheese then garnish with lots of kale.

Add salt and oregano

Broil for approximately 5 minutes (until cheese melts).

10 Great Kale Recipes: Soup

The dark leafy green vegetable is making fine cuisine taste even better. Kale is a Superfood packed with vitamins and fiber. Improve your health and your appearance with Kale Soup Recipes.

A one cup serving of kale contains RDA recommended nutrients:

2.5 g Protein
354% Vitamin A (beta-carotene)
89% Vitamin C
1328% Vitamin K
27% Manganese

Protect your cardio vascular system from heart disease. Also identified as a cancer fighting agent, Kale induces blood and bone regeneration. Balance your body with Kale Superfood Soups to beat chronic ailments. Kale assists the body in absorption of Calcium and Magnesium required for longevity. Ten (10) Delicious Kale Superfood Soup recipes can be prepared raw or cooked.

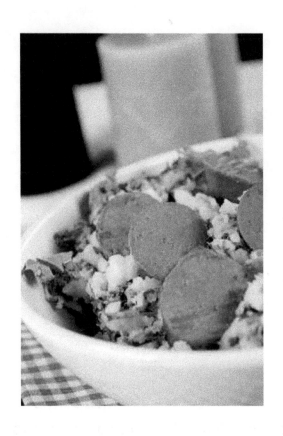

Kale Gazpacho

Summer Soup in Minutes

Ingredients

1 kale bun
1t olive oil
2 garlic cloves
1t salt

Directions

Toss cooked kale into a blender, add a little olive oil and salt, garlic and let chill. Add a lemon or lime for a fresh summer soup first or main course. Pour over BBQ meats. Kale Gazpacho is also great with cut vegetables or warm bread.

Dilled Kale, Beets and Tofu Soup

Rich Winter Soup

Ingredients

1 kale bun
1 bunch/can of beets
1 box of tofu
1 garlic clove
1t wine vinegar
Salt

Directions

Heat the olive oil in a frying pan over medium high heat.
The beets and tofu should be browned before turning
the heat down. When tender, add the kale, garlic, wine
vinegar, and salt and cook for to a bright green
consistency.

Cool. Add the mixture to the blender.

In the winter the soup can be poured as gravy over
mashed potatoes. Add 2T of olive oil, 2T of fresh dill
chopped, and salt to taste.

Kale and Bean Soup

A Whole Meal

Ingredients

1 canned or fresh cooked white beans
1 kale bun
1t olive oil
Salt

Directions

Heat the olive oil in a frying pan over medium high heat.
Add beans. Simmer. Turn down the heat and add the
kale. When tender, add salt and hot sauce.

Sri Lanka Kale Coconut Soup

Southeast Asian Flavor

Ingredients

1 chopped red onion
1 to 2 chopped hot chili peppers (remove seeds)
12 oz of thinly sliced kale (remove stems)
1/4 tsp ground cumin
1/2 cup shredded coconut, fresh or frozen
1 to 2 t of lime juice
Ground pepper
Salt to taste

Directions

Heat a large non-stick skillet and add the chopped
onions and peppers. Simmer. Add water sparingly to
avoid sticking. Once hot, add the kale and a 1/4 cup of
water, followed by the cumin and pepper seasoning. Stir
cooking for 4 to 5 minutes until the kale is wilted. Only
add water if more soup is desired. Finally, add the
coconut and 1 T of lime juice. Turn off the heat, salt to
taste. Serve hot or cold. Total preparation time: 10
minutes.

Sesame Noodle & Kale Soup

A Taste of the Orient

Ingredients

1 large bunch kale
3 teaspoons soy sauce
2 tablespoons sesame seeds
1 teaspoon brown sugar
1 teaspoon vinegar (rice wine)

Directions

Wash bunch of Kale, removing the thicker stems then cut the Kale into ribbons 1 cm long, place in a strainer and set aside. Sprinkle with 1T of salt and rub salt into the stalks.

In a small frying pan, toast the sesame seeds until golden brown over low heat. Add Kale and simmer. Cool and mix with the soy sauce, wine vinegar and brown sugar in a food processor or blender. Add water and reheat to boil. Add noodles. Salt the soup to taste.

Tuscan Kale Soup

A Taste of Italy

Ingredients

1 bun of kale
2t olive oil
2 cloves of garlic
1 box bowtie pasta
1 handful of rock salt

Directions

Heat olive oil, salt and garlic in a sauce pan. Add washed and cut kale to the oil. Simmer until limp. Remove from heat. Boil water, add rock salt. Cook bowtie pasta. Drain the pasta and add it to the kale mixture. Add ¼ cup of water and slightly boil.

Kale & Avocado Gazpacho

Green Goddess Raw Soup for the Soul

Ingredients

1 kale bun shredded
1 cup tomato chopped
1/2 avocado
1-2 t olive oil or hemp seed oil
1/2 lemon
Sea salt, to taste
1/8 tsp cayenne

Directions

Add olive oil to saucepan. Toss in salt while heating. Add kale and 1T of water. Cool. Add kale to blender with the remainder of the ingredients.

Serve with lemon.

Raw Kale Soup

A True Raw Concoction- Boost with Protein Powder

Ingredients

1 kale bun shredded
1 carrot
2t olive or sesame oil
2 garlic cloves
Salt
Protein powder (optional)

Directions

Blend shredded kale and carrot. Add olive oil, garlic and salt. Flavorless protein powder will enhance the power of your superfood soup. Drink up.

Sesame Kale Soup

An Oshitashi, Steamed Japanese Dish

Ingredients

1 kale bun
12 oz. soba, udon, fettuccine or spaghetti
2 t sesame oil (toasted) or additional for taste
2 t tamari or additional to taste
2 t black or white sesame seeds (toasted)

Directions

Place sliced kale into a pot of boiling water. Remove and wash again. Let water come to a boil once more then out in pasta and let cook until al dente. Add kale and cook uncovered over high heat. Drain pasta and kale and return to pot with sesame oil and tamari. Add sesame seeds and serve hot.

Green Power Soup

Kale and Broccoli Paired Up for Optimum Blood Efficiency

Ingredients

1 kale bun
1-2 large broccoli florets
2 t toasted sesame oil or to taste
2 t tamari or to taste
2 t toasted white or black sesame seeds

Directions

Place sliced broccoli and kale into a pot of salted boiling water then cook until wilted. Remove and cool. Place the greens in a food processor or blender with the sesame oil and tamari. Heat up or serve cold. Sprinkle sesame seeds on top.

10 Great Kale Recipes: Salads

Everyone knows that Kale is one of the best greens your body can consume. So why not use it as a replacement for other green dishes. Let's replace the romaine lettuce with fresh kale in our raw salads. The great thing about salads is that they are quick, easy, and convenient. Everybody loves something that they can throw together on the go. Kale can be a bit chewy so before you make a raw kale salad, considered massaging it a bit to soften it up, then enjoy. Here are a few great Kale salad ideas that your friends, family, and yourself can enjoy and make.

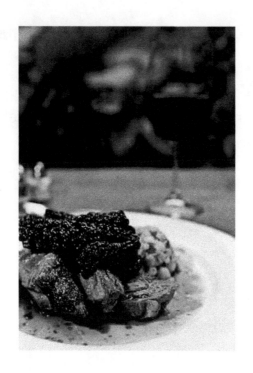

Kale Salad with Parmesan, Avocado and Apricots

Keep in mind this is a serving size for one, you can always add or remove any ingredients as preferred. Also add more for groups.

Ingredients

1/2 avocado
2 tablespoons vinegar (red wine)
1 tablespoon olive oil (extra-virgin)
8-10 flakes of cheese (Parmesan)
1/4 cup almonds
1/3 cup cooked beans
6-8 apricots (dried)
6-8 ounces of kale
Pepper and salt

Directions

Once you have your Kale go ahead and use tear into pieces using fingers. Remember to rip off the middle hard part of the kale. Make sure you tear them into bite size pieces and place into a medium size bowl.

Cut the apricots up into tiny pieces and put them in the bowl. Also throw in your beans, almonds, and cheese.

Stir together your vinegar and oil, and pour all over with a dash of salt.

Cube the avocados and put them all over salad. The salad can stay fresh for twenty-four hours.

Tuscan Kale Salad

This salad keeps it very simple. This is the ultimate raw kale salad. All you need to do is tear up your kale and throw it in a bowl. Put whatever dressing you would like over it but here is a recipe for a great Tuscan flavorful dressing.

Ingredients

Parmesan or Pecorino Cheese
Garlic
Red pepper flakes
Pepper and salt
Lemon juice
Olive oil

Directions

Mix altogether and let it sit on the kale for about 10-15 minutes, then serve.

Pickled Watermelon Radish with Kale Salad

Ingredients

1/4 cup toasted pumpkin seeds
Black pepper (freshly ground)
1 teaspoon thyme leaves (fresh)
1 teaspoon lemon juice
1 tablespoon pumpkin seed oil (toasted)
2 tablespoons olive oil (extra virgin)
1 bunch kale
1 watermelon radish (regular radishes can be used)
Kosher salt
1/4 cup sugar
1/2 cup vinegar (white wine)

Directions

Combined salt, sugar and vinegar in a medium size bowl.
Slice the radish thinly and add to the bowl. Stir
everything together to make sure that the radish slices
are fully saturated. Let it stand for about 30 minutes.

Tear kale into bite size pieces. In a large bowl mix all
other ingredients - thyme, lemon juice, pumpkin seed oil
and olive oil. Add the kale into the bowl and massage
together. Drain the radishes and toss into the large

bowl. Use pumpkin seeds to garnish.

Kale Salad with Lemon and Pecorino

Ingredients

Fresh black pepper and Kosher salt (to taste)
1/2 cup olive oil
2 juiced lemons
4 ounces grated Pecorino Romano
1 big bunch kale washed and trim the stems off

Directions

Cut the kale into ribbon length pieces. Toss the cheese together with kale. Stir together lemon juice and olive oil and pour over the salad. Season with salt and pepper then let stand for about an hour prior to serving.

Kale Salad with Meyer Lemon and Blood Orange

Ingredients

Freshly ground black pepper and kosher salt
1/4 cup olive oil (extra-virgin)
1 large finely chopped shallot
Zest of 1 Meyer lemon
4 small segmented blood oranges (reserve the juice)
1 bunch black kale

Directions

Wash and trim kale. Cut into ribbon sliced pieces.

In a large bowl mix together your black pepper, salt, olive oil, shallots, Meyer lemon zest and blood orange then put in the kale. Toss and let stand for about 20 minutes then season as desired.

Ricotta and Kale Salad

Ingredients

Ricotta
Pine Nuts
Shallots
Lemon Juice
Olive oil
Kale

Directions

Wash and trim your Kale. Tear into bite size pieces and throw into a medium size bowl. Cut up a brick of ricotta and place in the bowl with kale.

Mix together olive oil, lemon juice and shallots. Pour over your kale and massage together. Let it sit for a little bit and then top with pine nuts. Enjoy.

Kale Slaw with Peanut Dressing

Ingredients

1/2 teaspoon coarse salt

1 tablespoon packed light-brown sugar

3 tablespoons cider vinegar

1/3 cup vegetable oil

3/4 cup divided, roasted peanuts (salted)

1 large peeled carrot

2 red bell peppers clean then cut into fine strips

2 large bunches lacinato or curly kale

Pinch red pepper flakes (optional)

Directions

Finely chop your kale. Toss your kale with ½ cup peanuts, bell peppers, carrots, and red peppers.

Use a food processor to puree the rest of the peanuts with pepper and salt flakes, sugar, vinegar and oil.

Toss dressing in the bowl and let sit for a couple minutes prior to serving.

Mixed Kale Salad

Ingredients

Freshly ground black pepper to taste
1 teaspoon Dijon mustard
3 tablespoons freshly squeezed orange juice
2 tablespoons balsamic vinegar
2 tablespoons sunflower seeds
2 large mandarins (peel and cut in segments)
1/2 thinly sliced red pepper
1/2 red onion, sliced thinly
1/2 cup chopped red cabbage
1 cup chopped Tuscan kale
1 cup chopped purple kale

Directions

Mix the sunflower seeds, mandarins, red pepper, red cabbage, red onion, Tuscan kale and purple kale in a medium size bowl.

Mix together Dijon mustard, orange juice and balsamic vinegar.

Pour over the salad and toss. Season and serve.

Northern Spy Kale Salad

Ingredients

Pecorino or other hard cheese, for shaving (optional)
Fresh lemon juice
1/4 cup finely chopped or crumbled Cabot clothbound cheddar
1/4 cup almonds (cut in half)
1 bunch kale (remove ribs and slice thinly)
Freshly ground pepper and salt
Extra-virgin olive oil
1/2 cup cubed winter, butternut or kabocha squash

Directions

Trim and tear kale into a large bowl.

Cook Squash and cube, throw into bowl with the kale.

Mix all other
Ingredients
 in and top with cheese.

Kale Miso Salad with Tofu

Ingredients

2 cloves minced garlic

2 tablespoons miso

2 tablespoons lemon juice

14-ounce drained package extra-firm tofu

Directions

Preheat oven to 420 and coat tofu with the above ingredients.

Let cook for about 18-20 minutes then take out to cool.

10 Great Kale Recipes: Main Dishes

Kale and Sesame Noodles

Ingredients

1 large bunch of kale
12 oz of noodles (spaghetti, soba noodles or udon noodles can be used)
2 tablespoons sesame seeds (white or black)
Toasted sesame oil (to taste)
Tamari (to taste)

Directions

Bring a large pot of water to a boil. Cut off kale's stem. Slice kale leaves finely.

Rinse kale in large bowl to remove grit. Add pasta to large pot when water has come to a boil. Cook pasta five minutes less than directed.

Add kale to the large pot with pasta. Push leaves to

submerge in water.

Cook uncovered on high for five minutes or until both kale and pasta are tender.

Drain then add sesame oil and tamari to taste.

Toss in sesame seeds and serve.

Kale and Scallion Fried Rice

Ingredients

1 large bunch of kale
2 ½ cups of brown rice
3 large scallions
2 garlic cloves
1 ½ tablespoons of vegetable oil
1 tablespoon of soy sauce

Directions

Slice kale leaves and steam for 8 minutes. Cut scallions in 1/8 inch slices.

Peel and mince garlic cloves. Rinse rice thoroughly. Add rice into a pot with 4 ¼ cups of water. Bring to a simmer and cook for about 40 minutes. Strain rice.

On medium low heat, heat vegetable oil in a saucepan. Add garlic and cook for 2 minutes (do not brown garlic). Increase heat to medium and add kale and scallions. Cook for two minutes or so. Add rice and cook for two more minutes. Stir. Add soy sauce and stir.

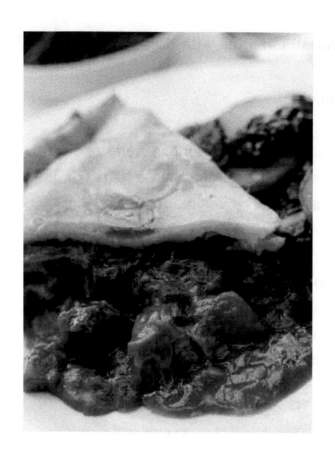

Vegetarian Lasagna with Kale

Ingredients

1 lb of kale (wash, dry, remove stems and slice)
8 oz shredded mozzarella cheese (part skim)
9 lasagna noodles (oven ready)
.8 oz white sauce mix
1 tablespoon of minced garlic
Cherry or grape tomatoes (halved)
5 oz ricotta cheese
1 teaspoon olive oil
4 cups of sliced onions
Salt
Pepper

Directions

Prepare white sauce mix by following directions on packet. Heat vegetable oil in saucepan and sauté onion until golden in color. Add kale and pepper. Cook until wilted. Add a thin layer of white sauce to a baking dish.

Top with three lasagna noodles (do not overlap). Spread with ricotta cheese then layer with tomatoes, kale and sauce. Sprinkle with mozzarella cheese. Repeat once.

Top with remaining 3 lasagna noodles and cover with remaining white sauce and mozzarella cheese. Cover and bake at 375 degrees for 50 minutes.

Cajun Chicken Skillet with Kale

Ingredients

8 chicken drumsticks (skinless)
8 ounces of kielbasa sausage (cut into small bits)
1 lb of kale (remove stems and chop leaves
2 cups chicken broth
1 cup white rice (uncooked, converted)
4 teaspoons vegetable oil
1 tablespoon of cider vinegar
½ teaspoon of hot sauce
1 onion (chopped)
1 red bell pepper (cut into strips)

Directions

Heat 2 teaspoon of oil in a large nonstick skillet. Add drumsticks and cover. Turn occasionally. Cook until slightly brown. Remove from skillet and transfer to plate.

Heat remaining vegetable oil. Add bell pepper and onions. Cook until translucent. Add kale in smaller batches. When previous batch cooks down, continue to add more. Add rice and chicken broth. Stir. Place chicken on top. Add kielbasa. Stir

Cover and simmer for ten minutes. Cook until rice is tender, broth is absorbed and chicken is fully cooked. Finish off with hot sauce and cider vinegar.

Kale and Spinach Turnover

Ingredients

3 cups of kale (chopped)
1 can of refrigerated dinner roll dough
6 ounces of baby spinach (fresh)
3 ounces of crumbled feta cheese
2 ½ tablespoons grated parmesan cheese
1/8 teaspoon nutmeg (ground)
Salt
Pepper
1 clove chopped garlic
1 onion (chopped)
2 teaspoon of olive oil

Directions

Preheat the oven to 375 degrees. Heat oil in big skillet over medium flame then sauté onions or 10 minutes and put in garlic and sauté for two minutes.

Add kale and spinach and cook until tender. Add nutmeg, pepper and salt. Mix in feta cheese.

Cut dough into about 8 pieces then roll out dough into a circle 5 inches in diameter) then spoon approximately

1/3 cup of kale and spinach mixture onto the dough.

Fold over and crimp edges. Lightly coat with cooking spray and sprinkle with parmesan. Bake until golden.

Braised Chicken with Kale

Ingredients

4 skinless chicken quarters (leg)
1.1 oz flour (all purpose)
2 tablespoons canola oil
5 chopped garlic cloves
1 can fire roasted tomatoes (salt free)
16 oz kale (pre-washed)
1 can chicken broth (low sodium)
1 tablespoon vinegar (red wine)
Salt
Pepper

Directions

Preheat the oven to 350 degrees. Heat pan on medium flame then put in canola oil. Season chicken with salt and pepper then dredge in flour.

Place in pan and let cook for 2 ½ minutes on either side then remove it and add rest of oil to pan and add garlic and let cook for approximately 20 seconds.

Put in half of kale then let cook for about 2 minutes. Put in rest of kale. Cook for 3 minutes.

Add broth and tomatoes. Stir and bring to a boil. Add chicken to mixture and bake for one hour. Remove chicken. Add vinegar to kale mixture then serve.

White Bean Soup with Chorizo and Kale

Ingredients

2 oz chorizo (Spanish)
4 cups kale (chopped)
3 cup low sodium chicken broth
1 cup chopped onions
2 cans cannellini beans
3 minced garlic cloves
Black pepper

Directions

Heat large saucepan over medium flame then sauté chorizo for one minute and add onion and garlic. Cook until tender. Microwave both, for three minutes on high setting.

Add broth to pan and bring to a boil. Mash beans. Add kale and pepper to pan. Cook for 6 minutes. Serve.

Other great kale recipes include Cajun steak frites with kale, green lentil curry with kale and garbanzo beans with greens. All of these recipes are truly delicious, healthy and easy to make.

Kale with Steamed Halibut and Walnuts

Ingredients

1 1/2 pounds kale (trim stems)
2 large minced garlic cloves
1/2 cup walnuts (chopped)
3 tablespoons unsalted butter
1 thinly sliced lemon
Black pepper and kosher salt
3 tablespoons olive oil
4 6-ounce halibut fillets (skinless)

Directions

Preheat the oven to 400 degrees. Use a tablespoon oil to coat both sides of fish then place in a roasting pan.

Season with ¼ teaspoon pepper and ½ teaspoon salt then put slices of lemon on top and let roast for about fifteen minutes (fish should be opaque).

In the meantime, melt 2 tablespoons butter in a big skillet over medium flame. Put in walnuts and brown, stirring often. When done, remove from skillet and place to one side.

Put in garlic and rest of butter and oil and let cook for ½ a minute.

Put in kale, ½ teaspoon salt and ½ cup water then toss. Cover and let cook for about five minutes until kale is wilted (toss often). Mix in the walnuts and serve with the fish.

Greens and Garbanzo Beans

Ingredients

1/2 cup plain Greek yogurt (2% reduced-fat)
4 cups fresh kale (chopped)
2 cans rinsed and drained garbanzo beans (organic chickpeas)
1 cup water
2 1/2 cups fat-free chicken broth (lower-sodium)
1/2 teaspoon red pepper (crushed)
1/2 teaspoon cumin (ground)
1/4 teaspoon kosher salt
1 teaspoon paprika
2 minced garlic cloves
1/2 cup onion (chopped)
1 cup carrots (chopped)
2 slices bacon (center-cut)
4 lemon wedges (optional)

Directions

Place bacon in Dutch oven to cook until crisp then use slotted spoon to remove bacon and crumble it. Put chopped onion and 1 cup carrot in pan and let cook for about four minutes, stirring often. Put in garlic and cook for another minute, mixing often. Put in red pepper, cumin, ¼ teaspoon salt and paprika and let cook for 30 seconds while stirring often. Mix in beans, 1 cup water and chicken broth and let come to a boil then lower heat and let simmer for another twenty minutes, stirring often.

To the bean mixture add 4 cups kale then cover and let simmer until kale becomes tender (about ten minutes). In four bowls ladle approximately 1 ¼ cup bean mix then place yogurt on top (2 tablespoons). Serve with lemon wedges and sprinkle with lemon wedges if desired.

Garlic-Roasted Kale

Ingredients

1 teaspoon sherry vinegar
10 ounces chopped kale (remove stems)
1 thinly sliced garlic clove
1/4 teaspoon kosher salt
3 1/2 teaspoons olive oil (extra-virgin)

Directions

In the lower third of the oven place the oven racks then preheat the oven to 425 degrees. Put a big jelly roll pan in the oven for about five minutes.

Mix olive oil, kosher salt, sliced garlic and chopped kale in a bowl, tossing to coat. Put kale mix on the hot pan using a silicone spatula to separate the leaves. Let bake for seven minutes at 425 degrees the stir the kale. Let bake until kale is tender and edges of leaf are crispy (about five minutes).

In a big bowl place the kale, then drizzle on the vinegar and toss to mix then serve.

10 Great Kale Recipes: Desserts

When it comes to desserts health really isn't the first thing to pop into your head. Kale has been introduced into many different dessert type dishes, giving you the satisfying feeling of eating right but getting the sugar tooth satisfied. Here are a few great recipes you might enjoy.

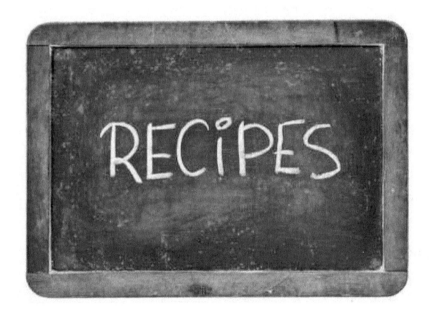

Coconut and Chocolate Kale Chips

Ingredients

1/2 tsp cinnamon
1 tsp vanilla extract
1/3 c cocoa powder
1/2 c maple syrup/honey/agave
1/2 c soaked cashews
1 bunch of kale (remove big stems and wash)
2 tbsp coconut oil (optional)
1/4 c coconut flakes (sweetened or unsweetened)
(optional)

Directions

Soak your cashews for about an hour in water. Mix the cashews and all other ingredients besides kale into a blender and mix until smooth.

Pour the mixed into a bowl over the kale until coated.

Move kale to a parchment line sheet and back in the oven at 300 degree for approximately 20 minutes. Flip them over and put back in oven for another 10 minutes.

Let cool, and enjoy

Bacon and Kale Bread Pudding

Ingredients

3/4 teaspoon pepper (freshly ground)
1 cup canned chicken broth (low sodium) or chicken
stock 1 tablespoon salt
2 cups half and half or heavy cream
2 cups milk
4 large lightly beaten eggs
1 1/2 baguettes (diced- 3/4-inch thick)
2 1/2 pounds coarsely chopped kale (discard tough ribs
and stems)
6 minced garlic cloves
3 finely chopped celery ribs
1 large finely chopped onion
1/2 pound sliced bacon (cut into ½ inch strips crosswise)

Directions

In a large skillet cook the bacon then put in celery and
onion and keep stirring until softened. Then put in the
garlic and the kale. Add into a bread bowl.

Preheat the oven to 350 degrees. Butter the dish. In a
large bowl mix together eggs, milk, cream, chicken stock,
and salt and pepper. Pour over the ingredients already

in the bread bowl.

Bake the bread pudding for about an hour. Let stand for about 20 minutes and serve.

Kale Cake

Ingredients

1 cup walnuts
2 cups of kale
1 teaspoon vanilla
1 cup oil
1 to 1½ cups sugar
¾ cup warm water
6 tablespoons flax seed meal
½ teaspoon salt
½ teaspoon nutmeg
1 teaspoon cinnamon
1½ teaspoons baking soda
1 teaspoon baking powder
2⅓ cups all-purpose flour

Directions

Preheat oven to 350 degrees. In a large bowl mix together all dry ingredients then add sugar and oil, vanilla, and shocked kale and stir until moist. Add Walnuts. Bake for about 18-20 minutes and let cool. Add preferred icing when cake is cool.

Pesto & Kale Muffins

Ingredients

1 tablespoon lemon juice
Freshly ground black pepper
1/2 cup olive oil (extra virgin)
1/2 pound chopped raw kale (remove stems)
1/4 cup Parmigiano-Reggiano
3 large cloves garlic (trim off end and peel)
1/2 cup almonds (chopped)
2 teaspoons kosher salt

Directions

Combine all ingredients in a food processor and mix until all ingredients are chopped.

Put into muffin tins and freeze.

Kale Colada

Ingredients

Non-Dairy Frozen Dessert
1/2 Cup Coconut Milk
1 Cup Curly, Dino or Lacinato Kale
1 Cup Frozen Pineapple Chunks
1 1/2 Cup Coconut Water

Directions

Blend on a high speed until combined then serve

Kale Cookies

Ingredients

1/2 teaspoon pure vanilla extract

1/3 cup unsweetened apple sauce

2 tablespoons unsweetened plain yogurt (almond, soy, cow, goat etc)

2 tablespoons flax seed (ground) - mix with 3 tablespoons water

1 tablespoon ground ginger

1/8 teaspoon salt

1 teaspoon baking powder

1/4 cup almonds (chopped)

1/4 cup mixed pumpkin seeds, dried cranberries and raisins

1 1/2 cups kale (cook in 1 tablespoon ghee)

1 cup brown rice flour

Directions

Preheat oven to 325 degrees, Mix ingredients together, place on a baking sheet.

Bake for 20 minutes

Kale, Pancetta Pie and Butternut Squash

Ingredients

1 ounce Parmigiano-Reggiano (finely grated)
8 (17- by 12-inch) phyllo sheets (if frozen thaw)
7 tablespoons melted unsalted butter
1/4 cup water
1 1/2 pounds coarsely chopped kale (remove center ribs and stems)
2 teaspoons fresh sage (finely chopped)
3 finely chopped garlic cloves
4 slices pancetta (1/8-inch-thick)
1 medium finely chopped onion
1/2 teaspoon black pepper
3/4 teaspoon salt
1 piece butternut squash
3 tablespoons olive oil

Directions

Preheat the oven to 425 degrees
Sauté the squash with salt and pepper until brown
Then cook sage, garlic, pepper, salt, pancetta and onion stirring often. Stir in water abs kale and cover and let cook (stir occasionally).

Place mixture into shell. Spread the squash and cheese evenly over the kale mixture. Place in oven for about 20 to 25 minutes or until golden and enjoy.

Parmesan and Kale Scones

Ingredients

1 egg
3/4 cup buttermilk (whole)
1/2 cup Parmesan (grated)
1/2 cup cold butter, cut into small cubes
1 teaspoon baking soda
1/2 teaspoon salt
1 1/2 teaspoons baking powder
3 tablespoons sugar
2 1/2 cups flour (all-purpose)

Directions

Preheat oven to 425 degrees.

Combine salt, baking soda, baking powder, sugar and flour in a bowl then put in cubed butter and mix in Parmesan

In another bowl mix egg and buttermilk then start mixing in kale and keep stirring until it becomes dough, knead and flatten into 1-inch disks and cut into wedges.

Stir until the dough is properly combined. Place dough

out onto a surface that is lightly floured and knead briefly. Flatten dough into a 1-inch disk and cut into 8 wedges. Brush with butter and cook until golden.

Blueberry Kale Ice Cream

Ingredients

1/4 cup almond milk (add more if required)
5-10 pieces pineapple (frozen)
1 handful kale
1/2 cup blueberries (frozen)
1 banana (frozen)

Directions

Blend all ingredients together in a high speed blender until thoroughly blended and serve.

Apple & Kale Muffins

Ingredients

½ cup chopped seeds or nuts
2/3 cup golden raisins
3 cups flour
1 tablespoon cinnamon
½ teaspoon salt
2 teaspoons baking soda
3/4 cup sugar
4 eggs
1 8 ounce container cream cheese (vegan)
Peel of 1 lemon
3 granny smith apples
1 small bunch kale

Directions

Preheat the oven to 350 degrees. Blend all the ingredients until smooth then pour batter into muffin pans then bake for 45 minutes.

Section 2: Smoothie Basics and You

What is a smoothie? What makes it so much different from any other type of drink on the market? The biggest difference of course is that the smoothie is a blended drink, containing a number of different ingredients. While some smoothies are designed for taste, others are designed for health. Then again, you always have the in-between ground wherein you can have both taste AND health benefits!

Before you get started with your smoothing making adventure, it would be within your best interest to make sure you have the right tools on hand. The most common items you are going to need, and find in common with all of the recipes in this book, is a blender. While most smoothies can be made with any blender, you will need to make sure you have a particularly high end one if you are going to be making vegetable smoothies. It can be a bit difficult to blend broccoli and carrots properly, and as you know, even a juicer might not get it right the first ten times.

A smoothie is comprised of a few different ingredients,

and once you look over the recipes named in this book, you might even try experimenting with a few of your own. The most important thing to remember however, is that while smoothies taste great, they are intended to sustain your health and even get you to a better place in your life. That being said, make sure you are using healthy ingredients, and most importantly, make sure you are using the right smoothie for the right occasion. Some are suitable for breakfast, some are great for lunches, and others are perfect for that energy boost you need first thing in the morning. Then again, some smoothies are better for the all important liver purge.

Common Smoothie Ingredients:

Chocolate
Peanut Butter
Fruit
Frozen Fruit
Crushed Ice
Honey
Syrup
Milk
Yogurt
Soy Milk
Whey Powder

Green Tea

Though these are some of the most common ingredients, we don't recommend that you add them all at once. Instead, we are going to provide you a few great recipes in the following categories:

Fruit smoothies

Green Smoothies

Breakfast Smoothies

Energy Smoothies

Before we get into the different smoothie recipes, let's talk a bit about the detox diet along with the function of the liver. Before you attempt to perform a liver detox however, it would be within your best interest to get to know the liver and understand just why it needs detox from time to time.

Liver Detox and You

Every system, whether organic or mechanical will need some type of filter. In the human body, the liver serves as the primary filter, and it is virtually impossible to maintain good health without it. The problem however is that we tend to abuse our 'filter' over time, and it will lead to some type of illness. If you want to stop this illness from occurring, there are a few things you need to do. First of all you need to make sure you remove all the excess fat from the liver. In addition to that, bile needs to flow free, and toxic waste must be filtered out. If possible, gallstones should be dissolved and passed while regenerating damaged cells.

Many people consider the liver to be the most important organ in the body, but when it comes to healthcare it is ironically forgotten. With 200 separate identified functions, the liver is vital for regulating and breaking down different substances inside the body. These functions include, but are not limited to the following:

Fat Storage Regulation
Blood Cleansing
Discharge of Waste
Energy Production

Hormone Balance

Tissue Regeneration(Self)

Storage of Vitamins and Minerals

Metabolize Alcohol

Manufacture New Proteins

Produce Immune Factors

Remove Bacteria from Blood Stream

Manage Chemicals

While the average person might not give the liver a second thought, there are many in the medical profession who are of the opinion that a great number of diseases can actually be prevented completely if the liver is in working order. An unhealthy liver will be like a gateway to all sort of disease and should be corrected as quickly as possible.

Harm can come to the liver in a number of different ways. One such event might involve an excess of protein in the diet, while you might also find that simple carbohydrates do their share of harm. The more fat you have stored in the liver, the harder it is for the liver to actually function. This is something for you to think about the next time you choose to eat an entire plate of fried chicken.

Overeating is another issue and serious temptation that

we all face. Not only is overeating hard on the figure, it also provides too much enzyme deficient food and stresses the liver. One thing that pharmaceutical companies likely won't tell you is that drug residue is typically left in the body after medications have been taken. This of course is second only to the inflammation caused by alcohol and other chemicals. The icing on the cake is a lack of exercise, which forces the liver to do elimination work typically performed by the skin and lungs.

Some of the most common problems in the liver can include digestive problems, constipation, low energy output, hay fever, diabetes, obesity, and even hypertension. As you can see, these are issues that you really want to avoid! But what do you do about it? The liver, fortunately, is an organ that is more than capable of repairing itself if you give it a chance. In spite of this, you need to do your best to keep healthy, and ensure that your liver is capable of functioning normally.

How do you know what sort of diet to use? As a rule, you should try to diet depending on the severity of the illness you are facing. In other words, the sicker you are, the more you need to clean up your diet. In any case, it is strongly recommended that you do a liver cleanse/detox at least three to four times per year. The smoothies listed in this ebook should give you some idea and perhaps even help you to start a healthier life.

Smoothies And Weight Loss

In the United States of America obesity is rampant -- this is an indisputable fact. With regulations being passed on food servings and the weight of the average school child skyrocketing, the need for action has never been more dire. Obesity can lead to heart disease among other rather nasty conditions, and with that being the case, many are turning to more alternative diets including the Atkins and Mediterranean. The problems with these diets have been kindly pointed out by nutritionists for years, though none so much as the Atkins diet. With the Atkins diet you will completely forego the inclusion of carbohydrates within your diet, and while this will eventually cause you to lose weight, you will find that it can have other side effects as well. As a matter of fact, many people have actually died using the Atkins diet! That being said, it is important to find a diet that will meet your needs without causing you to drop dead at work or at school. This is where the Smoothie Diet will come into play.

Why would you be able to lose more weight with smoothies than other diets? Many of them taste downright outstanding, and as you know, you can't lose weight with something that tastes good. The truth however is that a smoothie will give you all of the necessary nutrients in a single glass without the unnecessary calories. As you learn more about smoothies and study the ingredients you will find that you can build a great combination that balances protein, healthy fats, vitamins, nutrients, and complex carbohydrates.

Yes, smoothies can be designed to help you lose weight, but you may also find it necessary to develop one that boost your metabolic rate. This will of course involve providing you with more energy, and filling you up. Gaining energy in this manner will save you from needing to head to the store and grab one of those Five Hour Energy drinks. There is nothing quite like doing it naturally, and let's face it, Mother Nature has all the ingredients we require, and she is more than willing to cater to our needs if we just listen.

Benefits of Soy Milk

Throughout this e-Book you may see us refer to Soy Milk

or Almond Milk quite a bit. There is a reason for this! Soy milk is much healthier than regular milk, being naturally high in essential fatty acids, proteins, fiber, vitamins, and of course, minerals. These are the nutrients your body needs to function at maximum capacity, though you might be wondering exactly what Soy Milk can do for you in the long run.

The first thing that people will notice(if they are paying attention) is the improvement of their lipid profile. Unlike dairy milk, soy milk does not feature the same saturated fat or cholesterol. Soy milk is typically unsaturated, features no cholesterol, and is actually capable of inhibiting the transport of cholesterol into your bloodstream using the monounsaturated and polyunsaturated fatty acids. Regular intake of soy can actually lower triglycerides and LDL, or low density lipoproteins. If you have a history of heart disease in your family, soy milk might be the answer for you. In any case, it is always the answer when it comes to a proper smoothie weight loss diet.

What about blood vessel integrity? This is just as vital when it comes to basic survival, and it is another reason that we tend to include soy milk so often in our recipes. Soy contains omega-3 and omega-6 fatty acids along with phyto-antioxidants that will serve to protect your blood vessels from hemorrhage. These will also protect your lining cells from free radical attacks as well as cholesterol deposits. This is yet another reason why smoothies will help you lose weight AND keep your body in top shape.

Finally we have weight loss. That's why we're here, right? Though most people don't realize it, milk actually contains sugar by itself. Cow's milk contains 12 grams of sugar per cup, though soy milk only contains 7 grams per cup. Because soy milk only has 80 calories, it is the equivalent of skim milk. Through drinking soy milk you will gain extra fiber, and ultimately feel full for a longer period of time.

In a Nutshell:

Less Sugar than Cow Milk
Supports Blood Vessel Integrity
No Cholesterol
Inhibits Transport of Cholesterol to Bloodstream
Lowers Triglycerides and LDL
Encourages Weight Loss

In the end soy milk might be a bit more expensive than regular milk, but it will help you to feel fuller for longer, and will eventually drive your food costs down. In addition to that you will feel much healthier in the coming weeks.

Part 1: Fruit Smoothies

Fruit smoothies are not necessarily a health smoothie, though they do help individuals to lose weight. These smoothies do a great job of creating a meal replacement diet, ultimately giving you a tasty treat whenever you need one! Fruit smoothies are great for breakfast or for a quick snack at any point during the day. The best part is the way they fill you up. Rather than empty calories, fruit smoothies provide all the nutrients you require to keep you full and keep your hand out of the cookie jar. Each fruit smoothie will obviously consist of a base, and many people choose to use a banana. Others will opt for various flavors of yogurt, and in the end, it is totally up to you. You have so many different choices for bases and flavors, so go over the following recipes and see which suits you best for your day to day meal replacement!

Recipe #1. The Basic Fruit Smoothie:

What we have here is the basic fruit smoothie containing all of the ingredients you need to embark on your own sensational adventure in taste. From strawberries to chunked banana, you have all the essential fruits and more if you feel like experimenting!

Items Needed:

Blender or Smoothie Maker
Glasses

Ingredients:

1 Quart Hulled Strawberries
1 Chunked Banana
2 Peaches Pitted and Chunked
2 Cups of Ice (Small Chunks)
1 Cup of Orange, Peach, or Mango Juice

Preparation Instructions:

Place all of the fruit in a large blender, use the high setting until fruit is pureed. Once this is accomplished, add in your choice of orange, peach, or mango juice and continue blending until you achieve the consistency you want. Once completed, you may pour into glasses garnish with a slice of fruit and serve.

Note: Because this is the basic smoothie, you may feel free to try different ingredient combinations for different taste experiences.

Recipe #2: The Frozen Banana Smoothie

Though this is a smoothie of the frozen banana variety, banana will not be used as the base. Instead, lowfat Vanilla Yogurt will be used along with an amount of orange juice. All of the ingredients are fairly soft, meaning you can use a basic blender rather than a smoothie maker or juicer. This is one of the easiest smoothies to make so long as you have all of the ingredients on hand or can get to them easily.

Items Needed:

Blender or Smoothie Maker
Glasses

Ingredients:

1 Cup of Sliced Strawberries
1 6 oz cup of Lowfat Vanilla Yogurt
2 Frozen Bananas
2/3 Cup of Pulp-Free Orange Juice

Preparation Instructions:

Place the fruit ingredients into the blender on high and blend until fruit is pureed. Add yogurt pulsing it just enough to start the mixing process. Next pour in the juice and blend on medium until you reach the desired thickness. Pour into your glasses and serve.

Recipe #3: The Banana Berry Colada

Though you might not live near a beach, there is no reason you shouldn't be able to enjoy a tropical drink here and there – even if you're on a diet. This recipe brings the tropical island feel to you, and gives you the taste you crave without the alcoholic aftertaste.

Items Needed:

Blender or Smoothie Maker
Glasses

Ingredients:

3 Cups of Small Cubed Ice
1/2 Cup of Frozen Strawberries
1 Cup Pina Colada Mix
2 Whole Frozen Bananas
1/2 Cup of Yogurt

Preparation Instructions:

Layer all the ingredients in your blender and blend on high for about 80 to 90 seconds. Serve immediately.

Note: If you cannot find strawberries(they occasionally

go out of season) you can use strawberry syrup as a substitute.

Recipe #4: The Basic Grape Smoothie

For this recipe most people will actually recommend that you use red grapes, though to be perfectly honest you can use anything you want. Keep in mind that the ingredients mentioned make for a great smoothie, but you can replace the skim milk with regular milk, or the plain yogurt with low fat yogurt. Feel free to experiment and come up with the perfect combination for your needs.

Items Needed:

Blender or Smoothie Maker
Glasses

Ingredients:

2 Cups of Seedless Grapes of any color
1 Cup of Skim Milk
2 Tablespoons of Sugar
1 Cup of Plain Yogurt

Preparation Instructions:

Place grapes and sugar into the blender on medium and mix thoroughly. Add in the yogurt and blend for another

10 seconds on medium. Pour in the milk and blend on high. Proceed with this until the mixture is perfectly smooth.

Note: Though you are free to use any type of grape for this smoothie, it is recommended that you purchase a bushel of seedless grapes to avoid not having enough for everyone.

Recipe #5: Raspberry-Orange Smoothie

Orange is in fashion with this smoothie, but before you embark on this journey of taste, make sure you are actually using pulp free orange juice. In addition to that, you should of course make sure you are using ice cubes rather than chipped ice or straight water. The last thing you want to do is water down a tasty smoothie!

Items Needed:

Blender or Smoothie Maker
Glasses

Ingredients:

1 Cup Pulp Free Orange Juice
1 Cup of Raspberries
1/2 Cup of Plain Yogurt
2 Cup Sugar
1 Cup of Small Cube Ice
1 Sprig of Mint for garnish

Preparation Instructions:

Place your orange juice, raspberries, and sugar into your blender, mix on medium for 60 seconds. Add in the yogurt and blend for another 30 seconds. Toss in your ice and blend on high until you have the thickness desired. Pour into your glasses, garnish with a sprig of mint and serve.

Recipe #6: Kiwi-Apple Smoothie

If you're ready for something tasty then you've come to the right place. This mixture of fruits and vegetables might as well be a taste of heaven, and the best part is you can choose which leafy greens you want to include in your new concoction. Then again, you are free to experiment and remove the greens entirely! Remember – the smoothie is your oyster!

Items Needed:

Blender or Smoothie Maker
Glasses

Ingredients:

2 Kiwi Fruit Peeled
2 Apples Peeled and Cored
2 Cups Leafy Greens
1 Full Size Carrot
1/2 Cup of Water

Preparation Instructions:

Place the carrots and apples into the blender, pulse until small enough pieces to place the blender on high for another 60 seconds. Put in the leafy greens and water, blend on high for 30 seconds. Then add in the kiwis. Blend again on high until your desired thickness. Garnish with a slice of kiwi fruit if desired and serve.

Note: The leafy green may be lettuce or spinach. Baby spinach is recommended.

Recipe #7: Apple-Lemon Smoothie

Are you ready to try something sweet and sour? You've come to the right page! For this one all you need are a few ingredients and a bit of imagination. It's time to give your taste buds an experience that they will never forget, at least until you drink your next cup of hot coffee.

Items Needed:

Blender or Smoothie Maker
Glasses

Ingredients:

2 Apples (Any variety)
1 Full Sized Carrot
1/2 Cup of Water
2 Cups of Leafy Greens

Preparation Instructions:

Clean and peel your carrot, leaving one peel for garnish. Then slice the remaining it into small chunks. Core and cube your apples. Toss your carrots it into the blender. Pulse a few times and then add in the apples and water.

Keep pulsing until partially smooth. Add in your leafy greens, and put the blender on high until the desired consistency is reached. Pour into a glass and garnish with a strip of carrot on top.

Note: The leafy green may be lettuce or spinach. Baby spinach is recommended. It is also important to remember that apple skin must be left intact. While the apple should be ripe, it should not be brown on the interior or close to rotten. The skin of the apple contains plenty of nutrients and will help contribute to a healthy diet. That being said, choose your apples carefully and make sure you are using the same two apples in your smoothie. For example if you use a Gala apple, use two Galas, or if you use a Red Delicious, make sure the other is Red Delicious as well. The result will be a delicious meal replacement snack!

Recipe #8: Pear-Nut Smoothie

This recipe, unlike some of the others we have mentioned previously actually uses water as a base rather than yogurt or banana, even though banana is used as a core ingredient in this recipe. Keep in mind that you are using a peeled, frozen banana in this recipe, so it might be a good idea to invest in a high end blender or a smoothie maker not only to ensure that there is no damage to the device, but also to ensure that you achieve a perfect mixture. In addition to that, it may be helpful to acquire a glass blender container as these tend to be tougher.

Items Needed:

Blender or Smoothie Maker
Glasses

Ingredients:

1 Frozen and Peeled Banana
1/4 Cup Raw nuts
2 pears cored
1/2 Cup of Water
12 Ice Cubes

Preparation Instructions:

Pour water into your blender. Start layering your ingredients with the nuts on bottom, pears and ice in the middle and the bananas on top. Blend on low speed for 20 seconds. Increase to high speed until drink becomes smooth.

Recipe #9: Nutty Creamy Apple Smoothie

If you're not allergic to nuts then you might find this smoothie agreeable to your pallet. If you are, then you can always remove the nuts. Keep in mind that this recipe uses both water and yogurt as the base, making it a rather unique concoction. If you find that you do not like the consistency, you are always free to change it and experiment with different mixtures.

Items Needed:

Blender or Smoothie Maker
Glasses

Ingredients:

1 Banana, Peeled/Frozen
1/4 Cup Raw nuts
2 apples cored
1/2 Cup of Water
6 oz Plain Yogurt
12 Ice Cubes

Preparation Instructions:

Pour water into blender, layer the ingredients with the

nuts on the bottom, apples and ice in the middle and the banana and yogurt on top. Blend on low speed for 20 seconds. Increase to high speed until drink becomes smooth.

Recipe #10: Apple-Blueberry Smoothie

Apple and Blueberry are not typically seen together outside of a pancake or waffle setting, but they make fro a great smoothie along with avocado and leafy greens. You would do well to give this smoothie a try and augment your diet!

Items Needed:

Blender or Smoothie Maker
Glasses

Ingredients:

1 Cup of Blueberries
1 Apple
2 Cups of Leafy Greens
¼ Cup of Avocado
½ Cup of Water

Preparation Instructions:

Peel and remove the pit on the avocado then remove the core on the apple and cube bothe fruits. Pour the water into the blender, then toss in your apple. Pulse a few times to help break it down then add in the rest of your ingredients. Blend on medium for 30 seconds, then on high until you reach the desired consistency. Pour into your glass and top with one whole blueberry then serve.

Recipe #11: Cherry Apple Smoothie

Cherries and apples are always going to be popular. After all, they taste pretty great, don't they? This smoothie combines the two along with leafy greens, though as always, you may feel free to remove the leafy greens and make it exclusively fruit.

Items Needed:

Blender or Smoothie Maker
Glasses

Ingredients:

1 Cup cherries
1 Whole apple
2 Cups of fresh Leafy Green
½ Cup of Pure Water

Preparation Instructions:

Remove the stems and seeds from the cherries. Then core and cube your apple. In your blender add in your water and apple. Pulse these two items together for 30 seconds. Next add in the rest of your ingredients and blend on high until the smoothie is of the desired thickness. Pour into a glass and serve.

Recipe #12: CranBananaSmoothie

Though this smoothie might be filled with leafy greens, it is still not considered a green smoothie. By adding ½ cup of cranberries and a banana, we are creating what might be one of the healthiest and tastiest smoothies out there. That being said, you will most certainly want to put this one to the test as soon as you get the chance. Be warned that this DOES use water as a base, and therefore might not be quite as thick as most would prefer.

Items Needed:

Blender or Smoothie Maker
Glasses

Ingredients:

1/2 cup cranberries
1 Banana
2 cups fresh Leafy Greens
1 stalk of organic celery
3 Dates for Sweetening Purposes
4-6 Ounces of Water

Preparation Instructions:

Place the celery and water into your blender pulse 10 times to start breaking it down. Then add in the leafy greens, pulsing another 10 times. Toss in all of the fruit and blend on medium until desired consistency is achieved. Pour into your glass and enjoy.

Recipe #13: Plum-Apple-LemonSmoothie

This is another recipe that uses water as a base, but there is nothing quite like a good plum. These fruits have an entirely different taste, and make an outstanding addition to any smoothie. Combined with lemon juice and apple, you know your taste buds are in for the ultimate treat.

Items Needed:

Blender or Smoothie Maker
Glasses

Ingredients:

1 Plum Deseeded
1 Apple Cored
½ Lemon juiced
2 Cups of fresh Baby Spinach
1 Medium Carrot, Chopped
1/2 cup water

Preparation Instructions:

Place the water and chopped carrot into the blender use pulse a few times to help to break down the carrot. Add in the apple and pulse another 10 times. Layer in the last of the ingredients and starting on low speed work your way up to high until smooth. Pour into a glass and enjoy.

Recipe #14: Plum-Banana Smoothie

Because this recipe does not actually call for a frozen banana, you can use one at room temperature, and you will be able to use a blender rather than a smoothie maker. As always, try to ensure that all of the fruit is deseeded and preferably ripened.

Items Needed:

Blender or Smoothie Maker
Glasses

Ingredients:

2 plums, deseeded
1 banana, peeled
2 cups fresh baby spinach (or other leafy green)
½ vine ripe tomato
1/2 – 1 cup water

Preparation Instructions:

Pour the water into the blender with the plumbs and tomato. Blend on the low setting for 30 seconds. Then add in the leafy greens and banana blending on high until well blended and you reach the thickness desired.

Recipe #15: Kiwi-Banana Smoothie

This is yet another recipe that makes use of bananas, though we also have kiwis in the mixture. It is important to ensure you have enough kiwis if you choose to use the baby variant. Ideally you would obtain full grown kiwis, but sometimes the store simply does not have them. Try to remember this when you are picking up your ingredients! Because the kiwi fruit will typically be peeled, it should not be too tough on your blender.

Items Needed:

Blender or Smoothie Maker
Glasses

Ingredients:

2 kiwi fruit
1 banana
2 cups fresh baby spinach (or other leafy green)
¼ avocado
1/2 cup water

Preparation Instructions:

Peel your kiwi fruit and banana. Peel and remove the pit

from your avocado. Layer all ingredients into your blender. Blend on high for at least 60 seconds. You may need longer to reach the desired consistency.

Recipe #16: Kiwi-Mint Smoothie

Who doesn't like the taste of mint? Mint is used in all sort of tasty snacks, and often combined with chocolate. In this case however, mint is being combined with kiwi, banana, and spinach leaves if you so desire. Keep in mind that you can always swap the spinach for another leafy green, or remove it completely if that sounds more desirable. This smoothie is in your hands, and in your blender.

Items Needed:

Blender or Smoothie Maker
Glasses

Ingredients:

2 kiwi fruit
1 banana
2 cups fresh baby spinach (or other leafy green)
4 mint leaves
1/2 cup water

Preparation Instructions:

Peel your kiwi fruit and banana, slicing them up. Save a

half of a slice of kiwi fruit for garnish. Layer all ingredients in the blender, and blend on high until smooth. Pour... Serve... Enjoy...

Recipe #17: Cantaloupe Strawberry Smoothie

This is yet another recipe that might not be for everyone, but it does provide a slightly different taste if you are tired of the same routine over and over again. Once again you may feel free to leave the spinach out if you feel like going full fruit.

Items Needed:

Blender
Glasses

Ingredients:

1/2 medium/large cantaloupe
1 cup organic strawberries
2 cups fresh organic baby spinach (or other leafy green)
1/4 cup filtered water if needed

Preparation Instructions:

Cut your cantaloupe in half, scooping out all of the seeds. Slice it into manageable sizes and then make cubes while still on the rind. Cut the cantaloupe from the rind. Remove the hull from your strawberries and the stems from your leafy greens if needed. Place all ingredients into the blender, and blend on high for about 60 seconds. Add the water and blend for another 30 seconds if needed for desired thickness.

Recipe #18: Cantaloupe-Apple Smoothie

When you're in the mood for something a little different, why not going the cantaloupe-apple route? This is an organic recipe and is highly recommended for those who are attempting to lose weight. As always, we recommend this smoothie for those who are seeking something a bit lighter than those typically made from yogurt.

Items Needed:

Blender or Smoothie Maker
Glasses

Ingredients:

— 1/2 medium/large cantaloupe
— 1 organic apple with skin
— 2 cups fresh organic baby spinach (or other leafy green)
— 1/4 cup filtered water if needed

Preparation Instructions:

Cut your cantaloupe in half, scooping out all of the seeds. Slice it into manageable sizes and then make cubes while still on the rind. Cut the cantaloupe from the rind. Core your apple and cube it as well. Place your apples in your blender and pulse 10 times so that they are starting to get smooth. Add in the cantaloupe and baby spinach. Blend on medium for 30 seconds, then add water if needed to help to smooth out your drink. Blend on high for another 30 seconds or more to get the consistency you desire.

Recipe #19: Pumpkin-Apple Smoothie w/ Cinnamon

Anyone who says pumpkins are only for Halloween has never bought one out of season and turned it into an epic smoothie. If you cannot find pumpkins in your area, you have the option of finding cooked or canned pumpkin at your local grocery store. Nothing tastes quite as good as the real thing of course, but with a smoothie like this, you may have to settle for 'as close as possible'. In spite of that, this is an amazing concoction that you simply will not want to miss!

Items Needed:

Blender
Glasses

Ingredients:

– 1 cup pumpkin (cooked, canned, or raw)
– 1 apple
– 1 banana
– dash of cinnamon (to taste)
– 2 cups or handfuls fresh baby spinach (optional, but recommended)
– 4-6 ounces of fresh water or pumpkin seed milk (or try coconut water)

Preparation Instructions:

Prepare your pumpkin if needed. Core and cube the apple, place in the blender with your liquid and pulse a few times to break it down. Peel your banana, then add it and the other ingredients to the blender. Blending on medium for 30 seconds, moving up to high until you reach the desired consistency. Pour, garnish, and serve.

Recipe #20: Basic Sweet Grapefruit

While most people do not associate the words 'grapefruit' and 'sweet', here we have an outstanding grapefruit smoothie that simply requires water and a banana for the base. As always the leafy greens are optional, unless of course you're in a spinach type of mood.

Items Needed:

Blender or Smoothie Maker
Glasses

Ingredients:

1 grapefruit
1 banana
2 cups fresh baby spinach (or other leafy green)
4 ounces of water

Preparation Instructions:

Peel your banana and grapefruit. Remove all seeds from the grapefruit. Layer your ingredients with the leafy greens on the bottom and the banana on top. Pour the water on top and blend on high for 60 seconds or longer to reach the desired consistency.

Recipe #21: Watermelon-Banana Smoothie

Like several other fruits we have mentioned in this article, watermelon are typically seasonal, though they are grown constantly in the more weather permitting parts of the world. When you are making your watermelon smoothie, it would be within your best interest to remove all the seeds, or purchase a seedless watermelon.

Items Needed:

Blender
Glasses

Ingredients:

2 cups seedless watermelon
1 whole banana
2 cups fresh baby spinach (or other leafy green)
1/2 cup water if needed

Preparation Instructions:

Place your leafy greens in your blender and press pulse 3 times to help to break down the fibers quickly. Place the remaining ingredients in the blend and blend on high for another 60 seconds. If you want the smoothie less thick add in the water and blend for another 30 to 60 seconds.

Recipe #22: Watermelon-Pear Smoothie

Once again we're dealing with a seedless watermelon(unless you want to use one of the seeded variety and pick the seeds out by yourself), and this time it is mixed with a pear! As you may already know, the pear happens to be one of the most incredible fruits on the face of the planet, and one that will need to be cored before use. The pear is a fairly soft fruit, and this means your smoothie will be ready within a matter of minutes. You may feel free to use either a smoothie maker or a blender for this endeavor.

Items Needed:

Blender or Smoothie Maker
Glasses

Ingredients:

2 cups seedless watermelon
1 pear
2 cups fresh baby spinach (or other leafy green)
½ cup water if needed

Preparation Instructions:

Remove the core and seeds on your pear. Place it and the leafy greens into the blender. Pulse 10 times, then add in your watermelon and blend on high for 60 seconds. Add water if needed to reach the desired consistency and blend for an additional 3 seconds. Serve and enjoy.

Recipe #23: Tangerine-Coconut Smoothie

If you're ready to move into the more exotic portion of the menu, then it's time to have a look at this amazing tangerine coconut concoction. As with all the other it stars a banana, but it also involves an amount of cocounut water. This is one fruit smoothie that you simply will not want to miss!

Items Needed:

Blender
Glasses

Ingredients:

2 tangerines, peeled and deseeded
1 young green or Thai coconut (meat)
1 banana (or 2 cups papaya, cubed)
2 cups fresh baby spinach (or other leafy green)
2 celery stalks (optional)
4-6 ounces of coconut water

Preparation Instructions:

Place the celery in the blender and pulse to start breaking it down. Place the tangerines in next and blend that on slow for another 30 seconds. Add in the last of the ingredients and blend them in for another 60 seconds. Serve and enjoy.

Recipe #24: Tangerine-Pineapple Smoothie

We've mentioned a lot of different great mixtures, but none quite as fun as the tangerine smoothie. When combined with pineapple, you will rather easily see that this is one of the greatest and healthiest smoothies in the fruit section. If you wish, you can replace the banana in this recipe with two cubes of papaya.

Items Needed:

Blender or Smoothie Maker
Glasses

Ingredients:

2 tangerines
2 cups pineapple
1 banana
2 stalks of celery
2 cups fresh baby spinach (or other leafy green)
4-6 ounces of water or tangerine juice

Preparation Instructions:

Place your celery in your blender and use pulse until everything is broken down. Peel and remove the seeds from your tangerine, add it into the blender using pulse a few more times. Add in the remainder of the ingredients and blend on high until everything is smooth and still thick.

Recipe #25: Pineapple-Vanilla Smoothie

For the first time we are going to discuss a vanilla smoothie, and vanilla does far more than simply add flavor. There are many studies proving that the scent of vanilla alone could assist those who are seeking to better themselves by losing weight. Naturally the details are still being investigated, and those who do take advantage of it will still nee to get plenty of exercise. In spite of this, it is still a great weight loss supplement and something to keep in mind when you start dieting.

Another respectable property of vanilla is the way that it manages to reduce both stress and anxiety. A number of studies have shown it relives these conditions which has quite a bit to do with the scent. It has long been recommended that those suffering from stress or anxiety simply sip water or milk mixed with a bit of vanilla extract. Not only would this help to get rid of the stress, but also other problems that may or may not be related to the stress your body is experiencing.

Items Needed:

Blender
Glasses

Ingredients:

1 cup pineapple
1 banana
1/2 vanilla bean (or more to add extra taste)
2 cups fresh baby spinach (or other leafy green)
1 celery stalk
1/2 – 1 cup water

Preparation Instructions:

Scrape the inside of the vanilla bean, and place what you have in the blender. Toss in your celery and pulse 30 times or until the celery is broken down. Then add in the pineapple pulsing another 3 times to start breaking it down. Add in the remaining ingredients, and blend on medium for another 60 seconds until you reach the consistency desired. Pour, garnish, and enjoy.

Part 2: Green Smoothies

What is the green smoothie exactly? How does it work? Why does it work? Why should you incorporate it into your everyday life? Believe it or not, many people are now taking part in the tradition we rather fondly refer to as the green smoothie with good reason. After all, more than a few people have lost up to 40 pounds, and some have actually managed to relive themselves of serious health problems simply by drinking a green smoothie every day as part of their meal plan. Before we discuss some of the better green smoothie recipes, let's talk about the health benefits that you are certain to encounter.

If you really want to lose weight, then you really need to make use of the green smoothie solution. These smoothies, like the others, will provide plenty of nutrition, minerals, vitamins, fiber, and of course healthy carbohydrates. These will all contribute to your eventual weight loss of course, and they will even help you to reduce your hunger pangs. At some point, most people experience fewer cravings for junk food and more cravings for healthy alternatives.

With that being said, it is no surprise that eating a

smoothie every single day will often end with an individual craving healthy foods, and will also result in them eating the recommended 5-9 services of fruit and vegetables each day. Keep in mind that the more fruits and vegetables you eat, the better chance you will stand of fighting cancer and other diseases. The greatest benefit of the green smoothie of course is the inclusion of fruit which serves to mask the taste of vegetables. This makes it very easy to consume the allotted amount and give you the healthy advantage you need.

While eating your fruits and vegetables is always recommended, it can be somewhat hard to digest them alone. By blending these ingredients you will bread down the cells of the plants and render them much easier to digest. The blender will actually maximize the delivery of nutrients to your body, and it is much more convenient than preparing a salad. When you are on the go, there is nothing quite as efficient as drinking your meal through a straw.

It is no surprise that green smoothies will be high in antioxidants as well as phytonutrients. This gives your body a great way to protect itself against disease, and a great way to boost your energy. These are natural, whole foods that will give you the energy you need to get through your day.

Why not simply drink juice or use a juicer rather than drinking smoothies all the time? The benefit of a smoothie, of course, is that your drink will use the whole fruit and vegetable. These are not processed or littered with preservatives. Instead, you have a drink that is high in both fiber and nutrition. If you want to increase your colon health and your health overall, this is the solution you've been looking for.

Once you take full advantage of the green smoothies, especially the ones we will mention in the next section, you will find that you even gain a clearer, more radiant exterior. Because smoothies are high in fiber, they eliminate toxins properly. This is yet another reason that smoothies are outstanding when it comes to cleansing the body. To reduce your craving for junk food and give yourself a great advantage, start looking over the available smoothie recipes and use them to your advantage!

Recipe #1: Banana-Papaya Smoothie

It's time to take a look at one of our simpler smoothies, which happens to be the Banana-Papaya. With just four ingredients and a lot of taste, you stand a great chance of cleansing your body and getting the daily energy you need.

Items Needed:

Blender or Smoothie Maker
Glasses

Ingredients:

1 Banana
1 Papaya
2 leaves Swiss Chard
2 cups water

Preparation Instructions:

Put your Swiss Chard into the blender and pulse 5 times to start breaking it down. Add in your papaya and blend on low for 30 seconds. Add in the banana and water, blend on high for another 60 seconds. Pour, garnish, serve, and enjoy.

Recipe #2: Dandelion Smoothie

It might sound a bit strange to some, but Dandelions tend to make some of the best smoothies, even if the color isn't actually green.

Items Needed:

Blender
Glasses

Ingredients:

Handful of Organic Dandelions
1 Banana
1 Pear
1 Mango
2 cups water

Preparation Instructions:

Peel the banana and mango, slicing both up. Remove the core and seeds from the pear. Toss the dandelions into the blender pulsing 3 times. Then add in the mango and pear pulsing an additional 10 times. Last place in the last few ingredients and blend on high for a final 60 seconds or until you reach the consistency desired. Pour, garnish, serve, and enjoy.

Recipe #3: Romaine Lettuce and Avocado Smoothie

For this one you are most definitely going to want a good blender, though the ingredients are not bound to be too harsh on the machine. The recipe uses water as a base, as most green smoothies tend to do.

Items Needed:

Blender
Glasses

Ingredients:

3 leaves of Romaine Lettuce
½ an Avocado
½ Fuji Apple
1 Banana
2 cups water

Preparation Instructions:

Make sure to blend the romaine lettuce before inserting the other ingredients. Once blended, proceed to do the same with the other ingredients for approximately 60 seconds. Pour, garnish, serve, and enjoy.

Recipe #4: Fuji-Apple Avocado Smoothie

The Fuji Apple is not something that you will find in nature – usually. Instead, ti is actually a fruit developed at a Tohoku research station in Japan. It was first brought to the market in 1962, and since then has been filling stomachs and serving as a staple in smoothies all over the world.

Items Needed:

Blender
Glasses

Ingredients:

5 leaves Purple Kale
½ Orange
½ Fuji Apple
Small piece of Ginger
½ an Avocado

Preparation Instructions:

Place all ingredients apart from the apple into your blender, pulse for 30 seconds. Place the apple inside and then pulse for another 30. Check to ensure the mixture is completed, then proceed to drink, or continue blending if not complete.

Recipe #5: Rainbow-Chard Smoothie

If you were looking for the ultimate in health drinks then congratulations, here it is. The rainbow-chard smoothie is obviously based on chard, a vegetable typically used in Mediterranean cooking. Chard leaves are usually green, but in the case of rainbow chard, the stalk is a different color. Chard is thought to be one of the healthiest vegetables in the world, having extremely nutritious leaves, and always available when you want to make something.

Items Needed:

Blender
Glasses

Ingredients:

1 cup frozen Strawberries
1 Banana
1 Mango
2 cups water
2 leaves Rainbow Chard

Preparation Instructions:

Peel the banana and mango, slicing them both up into smaller bits. Now you will want to layer the ingredients from hardest on the bottom to softest on the top. You will want your rainbow chard closer to the bottom to help break up the fibers. Top with the water and blend on high until you have reached the desired consistency.

Recipe #6: Spinach-Banana Smoothie

This is the ultimate in green smoothie recipes. It might not give you the ability to leap tall buildings or show off muscles on par with Popeye, but ti will keep you quite healthy, and it will give you something to talk about!

Items Needed:

Blender(or Smoothie Maker)
Glasses

Ingredients:
1 large handful of Spinach
1 Banana
1 cup frozen Strawberries
1 Orange
Small piece of Ginger
2 cups water

Preparation Instructions:

Peel your banana, and slice it up. Peel your ginger if not already done and grate that into the blender. Next put the spinach in the blender with the frozen strawberries and pulse 10 times. Add the last of the ingredients and blend on high until you reach the desired consistency.

Recipe #7: Young Coconut-Pineapple Smoothie

This recipe is not intended to serve quite as many as the others, but if you want to scale it up a bit, make sure you replace the ingredients listed with either larger quantities or larger items. Before doing so, keep in mind that by using a young coconut you will gain more Vitamin B6, niacin, and folic acid.

Items Needed:

Blender(or Smoothie Maker)
Glasses

Ingredients:

1 young Coconut
½ of a small Pineapple
½ Pear
5 Leaves of Romaine Lettuce

Preparation Instructions:

Remove the meat from the coconut, and put it off to the side. Remove the pineapple from the rind and slice that up into chunks. Remove the core and seeds on your pear, cubing that half right into the blender. Pulse these together 5 times. Add in the remainder of the ingredients into the blender and blend on medium until the desired consistency is reached.

Recipe #8: Red Lettuce and Raspberry Smoothie

Items Needed:

Blender(or Smoothie Maker)
Glasses

Ingredients:

1 cup frozen Raspberries
5 leaves Red Leaf Lettuce
1 Red Apple
1 Green Apple
½ of a small Pineapple
2 cups water

Preparation Instructions:

Remove the ride on your pineapple, and cube up the half that you need. Remove the core and the seeds from your apples also cubing them. Toss your frozen fruit and apples into your blender pulsing 10 times to start breaking them down. add in the lettuce and and blend on low for 15 seconds, then add in the pineapple and water blending an additional 60 seconds on medium or until you reach the desired consistency.

Recipe #9: Bell Pepper-Avocado Smoothie

Items Needed:

Blender(or Smoothie Maker)
Glasses

Ingredients:

1 large handful of Spinach
¾ of Orange Bell Pepper
½ an Avocado
3 cloves Garlic
2 Tomatoes
2 cups of water

Preparation Instructions:

Peel and grate your cloves of garlic directly into the blender. Slice up the bell pepper and remove the seeds. Cube the portion you are using into the blender. Peel the half of avocado and cube it up into the blender as well. Add in your spinach and then cut your tomatoes in half tossing them seeds and all into the blender. Top with the water then blend on high for 2 minutes or until you reach the desired consistency.

Recipe #10: Tomatocado

Items Needed:

Blender(or Smoothie Maker)
Glasses

Ingredients:

½ an Avocado
2 Tomatoes
Pinch of Cayenne Pepper
Pinch of Salt
½ of a Red Onion
1 Orange Bell Pepper
2 cups water

Preparation Instructions:

peel the half of avocado, and cube it into a bowl. Slice the tomatoes into quarters, and place those in the bowl with the avocado. Peel the onion and slice chunks into your blender. Cut the peper in half and remove the seeds, toss your slices into the blender as well. Place the water and seasoning into the blender. Pulse these together 10 times. Then add your moist ingredients and blend on medium until the desired consistency is reached.

Recipe #11: Red 'n Green

Items Needed:

Blender(or Smoothie Maker)
Glasses

Ingredients:

2 Bananas
3 pieces of Celery
1 head of Red Leaf Lettuce
2 cups water

Preparation Instructions:

Chop the celery up into chunks placing them into the blender. Slice the lettuce up into manageable chunks tossing them into the blender one at a time pulsing 5 times between each chunk. Once the lettuce is broken down some, add in the water and peeled banana. Blend on high for 2 minutes or until the desired consistency is reached.

Recipe #12: Celery-Banana Smoothie

Items Needed:

Blender(or Smoothie Maker)
Glasses

Ingredients:

2 Bananas
3 Pieces of Celery
1 Head of Red Leaf Lettuce
2 cups water

Preparation Instructions:

chunk the celery into the blender and pulse 10 times to start breaking it down. Add in the water and lettuce, blending on low for 20 seconds. Add in the bananas and blend on high until the desired consistency is reached.

Recipe #13: Kale-Banana Smoothie

Items Needed:

Blender(or Smoothie Maker)
Glasses

Ingredients:

2 Leaves Purple Kale
2 Leaves Collard Greens
2 Bananas
½ an Asian Pear
2 Cups water
1 Cup frozen Raspberries

Preparation Instructions:

Slice the pear in half and remove the seeds and core. Chunk it up into the blender adding the frozen raspberries and pulse 10 times. add the kale and collard greens, blending for 30 seconds on low. Add the water and bananas blending on high until the desired consistency is reached.

Recipe #14: Blueberry-Spinach Smoothie

Items Needed:

Blender(or Smoothie Maker)
Glasses

Ingredients:

1 cup frozen Blueberries
¼ pound Spinach
1 Orange
1 cup water

Preparation Instructions:

Peel your orange and remove all the seeds. Place the orange slices into the blender adding the frozen blueberries. Blend on low for 20 seconds. Add the spinach and water then blend on high until you reach the desired consistency.

Recipe #15: Lovely Tomato

Items Needed:

Blender(or Smoothie Maker)
Glasses

Ingredients:

4 Tomatoes
1 Red Bell Pepper
1 bunch Basil
½ an Avocado

Preparation Instructions:

Slice your pepper in half and remove the seeds. Cut it into strips into your blender. Slice your tomatoes in half over the blender tossing them in when done. Add in the basil and blend on low for 60 seconds. While that is blending, peel your avocado and cube it, placing the pieces into the blender. After the last ingredients are in the blender place it on high until the desired consistency is reached.

Recipe #16: Purple Rainbow

Items Needed:

Blender(or Smoothie Maker)
Glasses

Ingredients:

4 leaves Collard Greens
4 leaves Purple Kale
2 Leaves Rainbow Chard
1 Asian Pear
Piece of Ginger
1 Banana
1 cup frozen Blueberries
2 cups water.

Preparation Instructions:

Slice your pear in half, remove the core and seeds, then cube the pear. Add the water, frozen blueberries and pear into your blender on high for 30 seconds. Peel and grate the ginger into the blender. Add the chard, kale and greens and blend on high for another 60 seconds or until the desired consistency is reached.

Recipe #17: The Monster

Items Needed:

Blender(or Smoothie Maker)
Glasses

Ingredients:

1 banana, chunked
1 cup chopped frozen pineapple
1 pear, coarsely chopped
1 cup orange juice
3 cups baby spinach leaves
1 tbsp. honey
3 tbsp. ground flaxseed

Preparation Instructions:

Place ingredients in a blender, food processor, or smoothie maker. Puree until smooth. If mixture is not sweet enough, feel free to add more honey. When you are satisfied, serve.

Recipe #18: Basic Green Smoothie

Items Needed:

Blender(or Smoothie Maker)
Glasses

Ingredients:

1 Banana(Frozen)
3 Handfuls of spinach
2 tablespoons peanut butter
2 tablespoons cocoa powder
1 to 1-1/2 cups almond milk

Preparation Instructions:

Peel the banana and cut it into chunks. Place it at the bottom of the blender with the spinach. put the peanut butter and cocoa powder in next. Pulse these together 10 times. Then pour in the almond milk and blend on high until the desired thickness is reached.

Recipe #19: Green Grape Smoothie

Items Needed:

Blender(or Smoothie Maker)
Glasses

Ingredients:

2 Cups Red Seedless Grapes
1 Cup Packed Greens- I used lettuce but Kale and
Spinach are even better
1 Medium Pear
1/2 Cup Frozen Pumpkin Pureé
2 Tbsp. Avocado
3/4 Cup Coconut Water
Optional: Ice Cubes

Preparation Instructions:

Cut the pear in half and remove the core and seeds then
chop it into rough cubes. Remove the skin from the
avocado and place that in blender with the pear and the
greens. Blend on low for 30 seconds, add remaining
ingredients and blend on high for 60 seconds or until the
desired thickness.

Recipe #20: Pomegranate-Blueberry

Items Needed:

Blender(or Smoothie Maker)
Glasses

Ingredients:

1/4 cup fresh pomegranate juice or arils
1 oz (2 tablespoons) whole acai berry juice or 100 grams
of frozenacai berry puree*
2 cups frozen wild blueberries
2 organic bananas
4 ounces filtered water (optional if needed)

Preparation Instructions:

Peel the bananas and cut them into rough chunks. Place
all fruit into the blender and pulse 10 times to start
breaking it down. Then add your liquids and blend on
medium for 30 seconds. Turn to high until the desired
thickness is reached.

Recipe #21: Acai Special

Items Needed:

Blender(or Smoothie Maker)
Glasses

Ingredients:

1 3.5 ounce serving of frozen acai puree
1 to 2 sprigs of fresh mint (to taste)
2 bananas
1 cup organic red grapes
1 small head of organic romaine lettuce
2 ounces filtered water

Preparation Instructions:

Peel your bananas and cut into rough chunks. Place the lettuce in the blender with the water and pulse 10 times to start breaking it down. Add the grapes, mint and banana blend on high for 30 seconds. Add the frozen acai puree and blend on high for another 30 seconds, or until desired thickness is reached.

Recipe #22: Cucumber-Pear

Items Needed:

Blender(or Smoothie Maker)
Glasses

Ingredients:

1 English Cucumber (or seedless)
2 pears
2 cups fresh baby spinach (or other leafy green)
1/2 cup of water

Preparation Instructions:

Remove the core and seeds from the pear then cut it into rough chunks.

Place it in the blender with the water and spinach. Pulse 10 times to start breaking them down. Then peel the cucumber and cut it also into rough chunks. Place that into the blender and blend on high until the desired thickness is reached.

Recipe #23: Citrus Sweet Potato Smoothie

Items Needed:

Blender(or Smoothie Maker)
Glasses

Ingredients:
1 cup cooked and cooled sweet potato
2 oranges
1/4 teaspoon cinnamon

Preparation Instructions:

Remove the skins from the sweet potato while still warm but not hot. Let finish cooling. If you want them to cool faster, you can cube them now too. While they are cooling, peel your oranges and remove the seeds. Once the sweet potato is ready, place it in the blender with the orange and cinnamon. Bend on high until you have the desired thickness.

Recipe #24: Banana and Broccoli Smoothie

Items Needed:

Blender(or Smoothie Maker)
Glasses

Ingredients:
2 large bananas
2 cups frozen broccoli, chopped
4 ounces of filtered water

Preparation Instructions:

Place the broccoli into the blender with the water and blend on low while you are peeling the bananas. Stop the blender and drop in the bananas and blend on medium for 60 seconds. If not smooth put on high until desired consistency is achieved.

Recipe #25: Celery-Red Grape Smoothie

Items Needed:

Blender(or Smoothie Maker)
Glasses

Ingredients:

1 cup red grapes
1 small banana
2 medium stalk of celery
2 ounces of filtered water if needed

Preparation Instructions:

Chop the celery into 1 inch chunks, place them in the blender with the grapes. pulse 10 times then put on low while you are peeling and chunking your banana. Toss the banana into the blender with everything else and add the water at this time if you like. Blend on high until you reach the consistency desired.

Recipe #26: Mango-Tomato Smoothie

Items Needed:

Blender(or Smoothie Maker)
Glasses

Ingredients:

1 Mango, peeled and pitted
4 Ounces almond or soy milk
2 Campari tomatoes
1 Cup pineapple
1 Cup cilantro
3 Cups fresh baby spinach

Preparation Instructions:

Peel and pit your mango, ensuring that it is properly
sliced. Chop your tomatoes, pineapple, and baby
spinach. Once these things are done you may place your
ingredients in the blender, mix, and serve.

Part 3: Breakfast Smoothies

Recipe #1: Blueberry Banana

No matter who you are or how old you get, you always have time for a meal, or a meal replacement that involves blueberries and bananas!

Items Needed:

Blender(or Smoothie Maker)
Glasses

Ingredients:
1 cup frozen blueberries
1 banana
6 ounces plain nonfat plain yogurt
3/4 cup unsweetened almond milk
1 tablespoon ground flax seeds
1/2 cup ice cubes

Preparation Instructions:

Place ingredients in the blender and begin blending on low speed. Increase speed gradually until ingredients are smooth. Serve and drink.

Recipe #2: Oatmeal-Strawberry Smoothie

If you're a fan of strawberries or oatmeal, this is the perfect smoothie to meet the morning with. By adding a little bit of honey, was can enhance what might have otherwise been a rather dull breakfast!

Items Needed:

Blender(or Smoothie Maker)
Glasses

Ingredients:
3/4 cup soy milk
1/4 cup rolled oats
8 strawberries
1/4 teaspoon vanilla extract
1/2 banana
1 teaspoon honey

Preparation Instructions:

Blend all ingredients in a blender with a glass container, serve immediately, or later if you plan to cool them for a while.

Recipe #3: Basic Berry Smoothie

There is always plenty of reason to get back to the basics, and that is precisely what this smoothie attempts to achieve.

Items Needed:

Blender(or Smoothie Maker)
Glasses

Ingredients:

1/2 Cup of blueberries
1/2 Cup of strawberries
1/2 Cup of blackberries
1 Medium carrot
1 Cup low-fat milk
1 Cup pomegranate
2 Cups ice
Preparation Instructions:

Place the berries in the blender and pulse for about 20 seconds. Next, place the rest of the ingredients, including the milk(2%, skim, or soy is fine) and pulse again for 60 seconds. When the mix is done, feel free to pour and serve.

Recipe #4: Banana Crunch Smoothie

Going the completely smooth route is perfectly fine, but sometimes you need something with a bit of crunch to it. So, why not add a bit of granola to the mix?

Items Needed:

Blender(or Smoothie Maker)
Glasses

Ingredients:

1 banana
1 cup milk
2 Tbs. of honey or sugar-free honey substitute
1/2 cup granola
1/2 cup of ice

Preparation Instructions:

Blend the ingredients, ensuring that the granola is ground properly and the banana is well sliced. You may use any type of milk you choose, though most will use soy, almond, or skim. Proceed to grind ingredients until mostly smooth.

Recipe #5: Raspberry-Peach Smoothie

Items Needed:

Blender(or Smoothie Maker)
Glasses

Ingredients:

10 oz Frozen Raspberries
1 c Canned Peach Nectar
1/2 c Buttermilk
1 tb Honey

Preparation Instructions:

Thaw the frozen raspberries and cover them completely in syrup. Place ingredients in blender bowl or container, blend until smooth. Serve.

Recipe #6: Basic Protein Smoothie

Items Needed:

Blender(or Smoothie Maker)
Glasses

Ingredients:

1 Banana
2 Strawberries
1 Scoop protein powder
2 Tablespoons sugar or sugar substitute
1 Cup nonfat milk
3/4 cup ice

Preparation Instructions:

Chop banana into slices, then hull your strawberries, ensuring that there are no seeds left behind. Add all ingredients to blender and proceed to puree until mixture is smooth.

Recipe #7: Cherry Vanilla Smoothie

Items Needed:

Blender(or Smoothie Maker)
Glasses

Ingredients:

1 cup Frozen Cherries
1 cup Frozen Strawberries
1 Tbsp ground flax seed
2 small scoops fat free vanilla frozen yogurt
1/2 tsp vanilla extract
1 cup of 100% cranberry juice
1/4 tsp Cinnamon

Preparation Instructions:

Because all ingredients are small enough to place in the
blender, feel free to pour them in, using yogurt as your
base. Proceed to blend your ingredients until they are
fully mixed.

Recipe #8: Basic Apricot Breakfast Smoothie

Items Needed:

Blender(or Smoothie Maker)
Glasses

Ingredients:
1 cup canned apricot halves in light syrup
6 ice cubes
1 cup nonfat plain yogurt
3 tablespoons sugar

Preparation Instructions:

Pour canned apricots into blender along with syrup(in can). Pour in yogurt and ice cubes, top off with sugar. Blend until smooth and ready to eat.

Recipe #9: Pomegranite Smoothie

Items Needed:
Blender(or Smoothie Maker)
Glasses
Ingredients:

2 cups frozen mixed berries
1 cup pomegranate juice
1 medium banana
1/2 cup nonfat cottage cheese
1/2 cup water

Preparation Instructions:

Make sure your banana is properly diced and ready to insert into blender, then pour your boxes of pomegranite juice, along with cottage cheese into the blender. Finally, pour in the half cup of water and blend.

Recipe #10: Coffee-Banana Tofu Smoothie

Items Needed:

Blender(or Smoothie Maker)
Glasses

Ingredients:

1 1/4 cups milk
1/2 cup silken tofu,
1 ripe banana
1-2 tablespoons sugar
2 teaspoons instant coffee powder, preferably espresso
2 ice cubes

Preparation Instructions:

Dice banana and insert all ingredients into blender.
Puree until ready to serve.

Part 4: Energy Smoothies

If you visit any gas station, or the checkout line at virtually any grocery store, you are undoubtedly going to discover a plethora of energy drinks. Some of these work, some of them do not, and sometimes it can be difficult to determine which is which. What you can be sure of however, is that most of these are nowhere near the picture of health that a good smoothie will paint. This section will cover the different energy smoothies, but before we get started, let's discuss the primary ingredients and the benefit they can add for the average smoothie. Each ingredient has health benefits and can add that extra energy boost to your day whether you need it in the morning, the afternoon, or the late evening hours.

Blueberries -- In many of the smoothie recipes you will find blueberries, even in those that are not specifically designated as 'energy smoothies'. Blueberries happen to be high in antioxidants, fiber, and of course, water. The flavor they add to the average smoothie is undeniable, and the natural sugar will give you a healthy energy boost any time of the day. Combining them with other smoothie ingredients on this list will give you an even greater boost without the health risk we have long associated with the typical energy drink.

Coconut Water -- Many athletes have embraced the idea of coconut water for the post workout recovery. The substance contains electrolytes, and will therefore help to rehydrate your body. When you are just coming off of a workout sessions, you will generally have less energy due to dehydration -- becoming rehydrated will give you a rather impressive and useful energy boost.

Bananas -- Every smoothie needs some type of base, and most people will choose bananas. Not only are they easy to use, they also help to satisfy hunger pangs. In addition to that, bananas help to make your smoothie much more like a milkshake due to the thickness it adds.

Cinnamon -- Cinnamon will definitely add a slight increase in your energy as it is considered a warming herb. In addition to that, it tends to add amazing flavor.

Almonds -- For those who are interested in a rich nutty flavor, Almonds are without a doubt a great source of healthy fats, and if you want to avoid the nutty flavor, you could simply try almond butter. Either way, you will find that almonds add a great source of energy for the long day ahead.

Dark Chocolate -- Almost everyone craves chocolate at some point, and with that being the case, it is no surprise that so many people want to add dark chocolate to their energy smoothies. For obvious reasons dark chocolate will help you to gain energy for the day, and it also contains a great number of antioxidants.

Recipe #1: Basic Energy Smoothie

Items Needed:

Blender(or Smoothie Maker)
Glasses

Ingredients:

1 cup low-fat vanilla yogurt
3/4 cup low-fat milk
3/4 cup fiber rich oatmeal
1/2 grapefruit, juice of
1 whole tangerine (without skin)
1/2 banana
2 teaspoons peanut butter
2 tablespoons vanilla whey protein powder
1 tablespoon honey
4 ice cubes
Direction

Preparation Instructions:

As with any other smoothie recipe, make sure you dice the banana. In addition to that, make sure your yogurt and milk are placed into the blender and mixed until smooth.

Recipe #2: All Day Energy Smoothie

Items Needed:

Blender(or Smoothie Maker)
Glasses

Ingredients:

1 cup ice
1 cup soy milk
1/2 cup fat-free yogurt
3 strawberries
1 banana
1 cup blueberries
1 tablespoon nutritional yeast
1 teaspoon flaxseed oil
1 tablespoon honey

Preparation Instructions:

Core strawberries and ensure all seeds have been removed. Place all ingredients in blender and proceed to pulse for 90 seconds or until smooth.

Recipe #3: Blueberry-Soy Smoothie

Items Needed:

Blender(or Smoothie Maker)
Glasses

Ingredients:

1 cup vanilla soymilk
1 cup firm light tofu
3/4 cup fresh blueberries
2 scoops soy-protein powder
1 tsp almond extract

Preparation Instructions:

Pour soymilk into blender followed by the rest of the ingredients. Once ready, pulse for 45 seconds or until completely smooth. Serve and enjoy.

Recipe #4: Super Energy Smoothie

Items Needed:

Blender(or Smoothie Maker)
Glasses

Ingredients:

1/2 cup orange juice
4 to 6 strawberries
1/2 banana
1/4 cup silken tofu
1 tablespoon honey or sugar
6 ice cubes

Preparation Instructions:

Slice banana and hull strawberries, then blend all
ingredients, serve immediately.

Recipe #5: Cocoa-Peanut Butter Smoothie

Items Needed:

Blender(or Smoothie Maker)
Glasses

Ingredients:

Makes 2 servings
2 tbsp 100% pure cocoa powder
2 tbsp creamy natural peanut butter
1 medium ripe banana
8 oz non-fat vanilla (Greek) yogurt

Preparation Instructions:

Begin by pouring the peanut butter, cocoa powder, and Greek yogurt into the blender. Insert ice cubes and proceed to blend at high speed. One the ingredients are sufficiently blended, proceed to slice the banana, add into mixture, and re-blend. Eventually the mixture will become completely smooth, and at this point you may decide whether or not to add a dash of cinnamon. Pour into glasses and serve immediately.

The Five Day Meal Plan

While having the various recipes might be great, knowing what you can do with them will help you out even more. The following is a five day meal plan. Keep in mind that you can mix and match these for different weeks, and of course insert your own smoothie ideas. The future of taste is in your hands!

Breakfast: Start the week off by checking out recipe #5 under Energy Smoothies. There is nothing quite like an energy drink to start the day, especially one with cocoa powder. After the weekend, you need all the help you can get to start moving! If you feel you don't need an energy drink however, feel free to try one of the other fruit smoothies we mentioned.

Lunch: If you want to get off to a good mid-day, then you might want to look into one of the red lettuce smoothies. Not only are they tasty, they have plenty of nutritional value. There are many other green smoothies on the list, all of which make for a perfect meal replacement – a real winner if you happen to be on the move a lot!

Dinner: While the smoothie is a meal replacement, you

can feel free to mix it up a bit with a solid meal so long as you do not cancel out the effects of your smoothie diet.

Solid Meals

Meal 1: Herb Roasted Chicken

2 lbs. bone-in chicken parts, skin removed
4 cups baby carrots
2 large onions
1 tsp. chopped fresh rosemary
2 cups hot cooked brown rice
1/4 tsp. salt
1/8 tsp. black pepper

Oven Temp: 425 (Could vary depending on your Oven
Cook Time: 45 Minutes

Meal 2: Pan-Seared Beef
2 Tbsp. Butter or Spray Butter
1 lb. lean top sirloin steak
2 large shallots or 1 small onion, chopped
1/2 cup non alcoholic dry red wine (or stock)
1/2 cup fat free reduced sodium beef broth
4 medium baked potatoes
8 cups green beans, steamed

Oven Temp: Pan Fry over Medium Heat

Pesto Chicken

2 Tbsp. olive oil
4 boneless, skinless chicken breast halves
4 cups whole-wheat cooked couscous
8 cups steamed green beans
Pesto Sauce Mix

Grill or Boil

Meal 3:
Pasta Salad
8 ounces whole grain or regular bow tie pasta
6 Tbsp. Mayonaise
2 Tbsp. chopped fresh basil or 1 tsp. dried basil leaves
1 clove garlic, finely chopped
1/4 tsp. ground black pepper
2 cans of tuna packed in water, drained and flaked
1 lb frozen green beans, thawed
2 cups cherry tomatoes, quartered OR grape tomatoes, halved
1/3 cup chopped onion

These are three meals that stand entirely apart from

your smoothie diet. During the course of the week you will have the opportunity to experiment with a number of different meal replacement options, each of them being a great choice for any time of the day. While they may not seem like much, these smoothies will fill you up and keep you on the go 24/7.

Printed in the USA
CPSIA information can be obtained
at www.ICGtesting.com
LVHW021732290124
770250LV00009B/449